1976 - Growing Up Bipolar

Mark Fleming

Tartan Moon Publishing

1976 - Growing Up Bipolar

MARK FLEMING

Mark Fleming is a writer and musician from Edinburgh. Diagnosed with bipolar disorder in 1987, he spent the following years being treated for severe depression and its polar opposite, mania as an in-patient in the Royal Edinburgh Hospital, and as an outpatient. He was prescribed antipsychotic medication for the next 30 years. Writing and musical appreciation have been instrumental in his recovery and ongoing wellbeing.

1976 pans beyond Fleming's peak-bipolar spell (1987-1990), delving deeper into the psyche of a young man haunted by a tragic childhood incident that might well have triggered the chemical imbalances prompting future ill-health. Candid and disturbing, but also humorous, joyous, and overflowing with pop culture references, *1976* paints a vivid picture of growing up bipolar.

Mark Fleming has been published in *The Big Issue in Scotland*, *Scottish Child Magazine*, *Gorgie Dalry Gazette*, *Cutting*

Teeth, *Flamingo Scottish Short Stories 1995*, *The Picador Book of Contemporary Scottish Fiction*, *Shorts: the Macallan/ Scotland on Sunday Short Story Collection*, *The Herald*, laurahird.com, *The 404 Ink Magazine*, *The Point* (Scottish Association for Mental Heath), pulp.net, and *The Leither*. His bands have included The Seduced, 4 Minute Warning, Desperation a.m., Little Big Dig, The Axidents, and Noniconic.

Some names, identifying details, and situations have been changed to protect the privacy of individuals.

ACKNOWLEDGEMENTS

For Karen and Elise.

Thanks to:

Scottish Association for Mental Health, the Royal Edinburgh Hospital, Hibernian Historial Trust, and my editor, Anne Duffy.

I completed the first draft of *1976* on 14th December 2021, what would have been my father's 100th birthday.

~

1976 is partly based on my novel, *BrainBomb*. That title was inspired by 'Brain Bomb,' two minutes 40 seconds of glorious thrash by art/punk combo Punishment Of Luxury.

INTRODUCTION

BrainBomb

BrainBomb was a semi-autobiographical novel I wrote in 2009. I wanted to document my experiences of bipolar disorder, reflecting on the wise words of my family GP, Dr Patterson when he posed this question: the human brain is so complex, the biggest mystery isn't why people have mental breakdowns, it's why don't they have them more often?

I fell ill in the autumn of 1987, sinking into major depression, culminating in my being sectioned under the Mental Health (Scotland) Act 1984 after being admitted to the Intensive Psychiatric Care Unit (IPCU) at the Royal Edinburgh Hospital. The initial diagnosis was a schizophrenic episode, revised to manic depression. At that stage, this was the sole diagnosis, rather than bipolar disorder. But according to psychiatric professionals, around one-third of bipolar patients are diagnosed with major depression because the latter is more common, it is the most frequent symptom experienced by those with bipolar disorder, and the criteria to diagnose major depression is the same as that for depression in bipolar. Those who *are* considered bipolar commonly receive this diagnosis from their teens to early 20s. I was 25.

During the 'flipside' of bipolar depression – the medical term is mania – patients might be embarrassed about their behaviour and reluctant to seek help. Some see the dip in mood swings as a price worth paying when balanced with the blissful optimism and outbursts of creativity and refuse medication. Others attempt to self-medicate with recreational drugs. English writer and broadcaster Stephen Fry admitted using an inadvisable combination of uppers and downers (cocaine and alcohol) to combat his erratic mood swings, or what he referred to as 'controlling the weather in his mind.' When I was experiencing mania, I exhibited the classic symptom of denying I was even ill.

When my bipolar graph soared into uncontrollable euphoria, I was hospitalised again. Discharged in the summer of 1990, I was informed my condition would be managed, not cured. I remained under antipsychotic medication for decades.

Given the stigma surrounding mental health, I decided to put my struggles behind me. If anyone asked why I'd spent time in the 'Royal Ed,' I made vague noises about drying out. Alluding to a spell in rehab seemed preferable to admitting being locked up in an institution known as the Edinburgh Lunatic Asylum until 1922.

When I fell seriously ill in 1987, my late parents left GP consultations with paltry leaflets covering a topic so stigmatized they wouldn't have been confident broaching it with anyone.

Although mental health now permeates modern culture, featuring in song lyrics and drama plots (along with helplines in the credits), there are still backwards steps. Piers Morgan, with 7.9 million Twitter followers, recommended 'manning up' as a catchall solution to complicated and often debilitating issues unique to individuals. Jeremy Clarkson (7.7 million followers) has disparaged people suffering from depression by jibing about 'Johnny Suicide' interfering with train timetables.

Experiences should never be suppressed or regarded with shame or embarrassment. They should be acknowledged, the back stories shared. Being an outpatient shouldn't have resulted in my employer placing my post 'on extended probation' due to my 'condition.' Like everything from broken limbs to cancer, mental breakdowns are a fact of life.

Although my recovery from severe depression was instigated in the IPCU, today the psychiatric community is also focused on looking beyond the pejorative term 'mental illness,' where the onus to resolve the situation lies with nurses, doctors, and psychiatrists. Much as the expression is thrown around by the popular media – and there are noble sentiments about the need to 'de-stigmatise mental illness' – scientific research paints a more complex picture.

For instance, it is suggested that mental injury rather than illness would be the most objective way of describing post-traumatic stress disorder (PTSD). Despite misconceptions about PTSD primarily affecting war veterans, drug addiction, abusive relationships, and stressful childhoods are seen as risk factors for developing symptoms. Psychologists are studying how mental health can also be affected by environment and genetic coding.

I eventually decided to write *BrainBomb* after becoming compelled to describe my journey through the darkness, no matter how eccentric, disturbing, or self-destructive my behaviour was at the time. What emerged was an honest story, heartbreaking for my family, but life-affirming.

One of my most rewarding experiences has been sharing my work at public events. I've read excerpts from *BrainBomb* at a diverse range of outlets, from an Edinburgh Fringe Festival venue in Craigmillar to the Scottish Mental Health Arts and Film Festival at Glasgow's Mitchell Library, from community writing workshops to schools. I'm proud to have been invited to discuss the book and what inspired me to write it following a request by users of Saughton prison library, and inmates of Barlinnie prison. After my talk at the latter venue, I was interviewed for the Barlinnie prisoners' radio station, Barbed Wireless.

1976

In April 2018, my case was reviewed at Ballenden House, an outpatient mental health clinic on Edinburgh's Southside. Since my final discharge from the Royal Edinburgh Hospital 28 years before, treatment reviews at my GP's had been scant, the doctors sometimes having to check what their online information resources could tell them about lithium. Prolonged usage can have a detrimental impact on kidney, liver, and thyroid functions, as well as impair cognitive ability. So I made this appointment to discuss the possibility of an endpoint for my lithium treatment.

When I asked the psychiatrist about likely outcomes of going 'cold turkey,' she reiterated the warning that anyone ceasing long-term antipsychotic medication faces a journey into the unknown, with the potential to regress. But regarding my own circumstances, she also admitted to having a lack evidence of *any* outcome, actual or anecdotal. No one else on her register had been on lithium for so long.

I mentioned the recent quarterly check of lithium levels undertaken by a phlebotomist at my GP surgery indicating a slight deterioration of my kidney function. We agreed on a course of action to reduce my daily intake over a lengthy period, down to the minimal clinical level of 150 mg, before ceasing. I swallowed my final dose in 2020, 30 years after my first prescription as an inpatient when the dosage had been 1,500 mg.

The onset of COVID-19 presented huge challenges to every sector of society, not least the one in four who will experience a mental health problem in any year. But lockdown also gave me the opportunity to kick-start a project long on the backburner: revamping my bipolar life story.

BrainBomb was written while still heavily medicated, and with haste. One reviewer, Stuart Blackwood, provided a glowing description: "Fleming's debut novel is lurid. Set mainly in his home city of Edinburgh, it's a bang bang bang mish mash which steams along at a million miles an hour. The astonishing thing is that this novel is seventy thousand words. The pace is so ferocious that it reads more like twenty thousand. This feels like a debut novel, an outburst of pent-up energy and experience."

He also remarked on its stylistic resemblance to early punk fanzines, the jumbled thoughts and ideas tripping over each other in their eagerness to land on the printed page.

Irvine Welsh also read it, commenting in his inimitable style: "Enjoyed BrainBomb, great stuff, but it moves like a rocket and it's totally mashed my heid."

One reason for this intense narrative was that attempting to remember spells when my bipolar curve was at its lowest ebb often drew a complete blank. That 'mish mash' contained ambiguity and poetic license, with some incidents wavering between distortion or outright fabrication. I also resorted to a convenient writing schtick for filling the gaps: fantasy sequences (partially inspired by Billy Pilgrim's time-travelling escapades in Kurt Vonnegut's *Slaughterhouse-Five*!)

But requesting and receiving a copy of my psychiatric case file from the Scottish NHS opened a window into my breakdown. Every medical consultation, drug prescription, and proposed treatment (including electro-convulsive therapy) was revealed in stark typewriter print or handwritten script. Especially revealing were the nursing staff's exhaustive observations of an erratic patient during my spells in the IPCU and the open wards, representing a diary of my painstaking recovery.

As I commenced my extensive rewrite, what began to emerge was something completely different. What I was writing was far removed from a semi-autobiographical novel distorted by escapist fiction. It was an uncontrived memoir. Its title, *1976*, refers to a pivotal incident during my adolescence. If mental health issues can be traced to trauma experienced when your mind is still developing, affected by happenings with the potential to alter the wiring of the brain – mental injury – I believe there is a compelling argument that my chemical imbalances were set in motion one afternoon that summer.

1976 isn't linear and flashes back to key events. Nor does it prioritise my mental health diagnosis. Rather than fixating on psychosis, it's a memoir in a wider context, sometimes almost like a companion piece to *Big Gold Dream: The Sound of Young Scotland 1977-1985*, Grant McPhee's 2015 documentary about the nation's post-punk and indie scene. If this book is a rich and multi-layered banquet, here are some of the dishes of the day.

Aged 11, being mesmerised by the brash meld of loud guitars and glitzy outfits of David Bowie, Slade, Suzi Quatro, Sweet, Marc Bolan and T.Rex, Mott the Hoople, and all the other glam rockers on *Top of the Pops*, taping their hits on a tinny cassette player. Four years on, the cathartic effect of discovering The Clash, The Sex Pistols, The Fall, Wire, and John Peel sessions. Later, African guitar music. James Brown. Motown. Kraftwerk and Krautrock. Bowie, Iggy Pop, Brian Eno, and Roxy Music's back-catalogues. Hip-hop. The Stone Roses. House. Techno. Ambient music.

Playing guitar and keyboards in bands from the age of 17, culminating in appearances on BBC Radio 1, Radio Forth, Radio Scotland, and briefly and chaotically, *The Tube* on Channel 4. Rites of passage, from pre-youth club alcohol binges and first crushes to the emotional turmoil of first love. The routine of an insurance drone in the 1980s and a Scottish Government drone in the 1990s. Scottish and Irish history. The positives and negatives of Scottish football, from Archie Gemmill scoring against Holland when we defeated the World Cup runners-up in Argentina in 1978, to hooliganism, the poison of sectarianism, and Wallace Mercer's attempt to end Hibernian FC.

The main courses include near-death experiences and the unconditional love of family countering the rollercoastering nature of bipolar disorder.

CONTENTS

CONTENTS

CONTENTS

CONTENTS

1

999

November 1987

I'm shaking. My pulse is racing. I must go through with this. I just need a moment's courage. I have to clear my head of all the poisonous thoughts. The easiest way to achieve this is knocking myself out. When I emerge from the blackout, I'll have a bump. But the delusions will have stopped. I'll have knocked some sense into myself. Literally. I'll be sane again.

Snatching breaths, I step back to the window. Run. Diving towards the bedroom wall, I crumple to the floor. I pick myself up. Another attempt. I smack into the wall with greater force. My face takes the brunt of the impact. Blood splatters the white woodchip wallpaper. When I hit the deck, it feels like the whole house quakes.

My parents burst in. Raised voices talking over each other. Dad's Irish accent accentuated with anguish. Ignoring them,

I haul myself up. Glaring ahead. Stepping back. Blood weaves around my chin. I charge again. This time Dad blocks me.

My crazed mind is warning this remedy won't work if I'm impeded. I must be allowed to knock myself unconscious. A further delusion: there will only be three opportunities for this to work. I've already used up two.

I shriek until my throat aches. Imploring them not to touch me. They *must* let me do this. Dad throws his arms around my torso. I try wriggling free. Find myself fighting a losing battle to overcome his determined resolve. While we continue wrestling, I catch Mum's agonised features. I plead, *don't touch me, don't touch me,* again and again. Shrill. Hysterical. Struggling to extricate myself from the muscular grip.

Mum is in the living room now. Talking to someone. Her voice strains with trying to sound calm. Who else is in the house? What is she saying? I hear her stating our address. Repeating this.

Like a defeated wrestler in a remorseless hold and pinned to the canvas, my bruised features are buried in the carpet. A sideways glance reveals Dad has hunkered down. Sitting on me, his weight is preventing me from further self-harming.

Sometime later, the doorbell. Unfamiliar voices intrude. Gruff. Broad Edinburgh. Two police officers tower over me. Disjointed speech crackles in their walkie-talkies. A paramedic huddles close, tugging at my sleeve. I wince at a needle's prick.

Dad relinquishes his hold. More insistent limbs take over. Ensuring I remain immobile. Another ambulance man appears. Helps his colleague secure me in a straitjacket. They lift me onto a stretcher.

I manage a smile at Mum and Dad. Both their expressions are locked in despair. I gaze at the ceiling coasting above my head. Feel a gentle agitation as the uniformed men negotiate the stairs. One asks me to relax. Keeps using my name. They'll sort me in hospital. He's promised my mum.

The front door opens to a biting cold evening. An alarmed blackbird chirps in May Annandale's garden next door. My eyes are drawn to the ambulance parked in front of Dad's car. Inside, I'm buckled to a table. After the door slams and we take off, I notice a red light. Yet another delusion flickers. To-night, they're coming in bursts. If I can state its colour aloud, I'll wake from this weird dream. Everything will be back to normal. *Red*. That's all I have to say. Like a password.

My mouth forms the shape. I've been struck dumb. It's far easier to close my eyes. Surrender to this mysterious journey. My bones feel soft as marshmallows. I'm floating. Through this black Edinburgh night. Backwards. Edging ever closer to a waterfall.

High Church

May 1990

After going to bed around 3 a.m. I'm up again by 7 a.m. Emptying the remnants of a wine bottle, I finish writing the short story I started yesterday. Deciding my ending's rubbish, I tear the A4 sheets into shreds, tossing them into the air like confetti. Ten minutes later I'm piecing together the jigsaw of the destroyed manuscript, a task made thankless by my sluggish vision. I give up.

Rummaging through packets of photographs stuffed in a drawer, I unearth a photo of me from 1982. I'm going through my Mark E Smith fanboy phase, complete with a grey blazer, argyle pattern tank-top, and brothel-creepers. This was taken at a stag party for a colleague when I worked for Scottish Widows, my first full-time job after leaving Tynecastle High School.

I recall a muted affair, tequila slammers and ogling go-go dancers replaced by lukewarm pints of McEwan's Export and darts in a rugby social club. The first stag night in history to feature a game of dominos? The most raucous part of the long evening was when someone scrawled: *I SUCK KNOBS* on the prospective groom's Adidas T-shirt in chalk from the dartboard.

Struggling against the tremors coursing through my fingertips, I remove the other hard-partying insurance clerks to leave a gurning close-up of me. I pop this inside the letter I've composed to Cathy Dennis.

I'm in my mid-20s but like some starstruck kid, I've decided to send her fan mail. This hearkens back to my teens when corresponding with bands by post was a thing. I would exchange letters with members of Crass. Abbo, the singer of UK Decay. A friend, Laura was a pen pal of Mensi of Angelic Upstarts.

Cathy's breakthrough single, guest singing with *D Mob* on 'C'mon and Get My Love,' a poppy house hit that topped the US dance chart, might seem a guilty pleasure. But a defining tenet of any post-punk collection is eclecticism. Among my records, she's filed between The Dead Boys and Devo. Only Luddites would denigrate New Order for having left 'Ice Age' far behind and becoming so danceable.

It's down to biology, anyway. Cathy could be crooning Hebridean sea shanties for all I care. A bubbly stage persona and sultry looks are an irresistible combination. Also indicating approachability. She'll reply personally, enclosing a promo headshot. Signed. With X's. So, the main thrust of my message is suggesting she drops by when touring Scotland.

I'll invite her for drinks in my local, The Balmoral. When I usher her inside, I'll steer her away from the lads who congregate around the fireplace, openly rolling and smoking spliffs. Mostly ex-cons, any plainclothes cops or off-duty Saughton warders they recognise entering are announced with a series of differing whistles. The roasting can be corrosive. Recent sample dialogue: *You, you cunt, reneging on the fucking rounds. I'll chisel the fucking cunt out of you.* Cathy won't be fazed. She's from Norfolk. It'll sound like a foreign language.

Writing a letter to a pop star is by far the least outlandish of my planned activities. Forgetting to add a stamp as I poke the envelope into the post-box around the corner, I now make my way for St Mary's, the Episcopalian cathedral whose three tall Gothic spires dominate Edinburgh's West End.

I contemplate the reasons why people all over the globe gather at their respective places of worship: church, mosque, chapel, synagogue, temple, huggable trees. There are times calling for celebration, or simple thanks. There will be occasions when comfort is required after natural disasters referred to, with supreme irony, as Acts of God.

As I make my way inside the cavernous building to squeeze into a row five from the front, I accept I fall into none of these categories. Instead of utilising the moments before the service commences for introspection, I'm engrossed by the magnificent stained-glass windows capturing the sunlight, the gleaming silver crucifixes. I'm in awe of the lustrous symbols, icons, and gaudy trappings because I was brought up in the austere Church of Scotland. Sunday sessions during my childhood made watching paint dry seem a riveting alternative.

This lurid setting is also a Protestant church but Scottish Episcopalian. Allied to the Church of England with its archbishops and incense. Much 'higher' than anything I've experienced. It must be akin to being inside a Roman Catholic chapel. But I've targeted this cathedral for that reason. The atmosphere is much more intense than the stern services I recall from Sunday School press-ganging. This is churchgoing on acid.

School history lessons about the Reformation described how the semblance of freedom alluded to by this revolutionary new take on state religion defined Scotland as a nation, Presbyterian plainness a reaction to the corruption and hypocrisies of 16th-century Christendom. As for the Anglican thing, the reason everyone is here today can be traced back to England's King Henry VIII, spree killer of wives.

Requiring a quick divorce in 1527, when this was refused by Pope Clement, he started his own church. Already a paranoid narcissist, as England's answer to His Holiness, treason and heresy against his royal supremacy was heresy against God. During his bloodbath of a reign, he ignored the fifth commandment and saw to it that upwards of 50,000 of his subjects were executed as heretics. Including Anne Boleyn and Catherine Howard.

The origin of this religion I've infiltrated this morning is down to someone's sex life; specifically, the lack of the single gene present in the Y chromosome of Henry's spermatozoon when he impregnated Anne Boleyn: the tiny swimmer that would have granted him a coveted male heir.

Reformation sounds innocuous. Led Zeppelin reformed for Live Aid. But over the centuries, worshippers on either side of this schism in Christianity have found their respective journeys to meet the same Maker cut short by lethal sectarianism.

My freewheeling mind is now fixating on the arbitrary roulette wheel of life. One sperm differently programmed at that moment inside Klara Hitler or Keke Stalin would have prevented millions of deaths.

As one christened into the Scottish 'Kirk', I feel like a Trotskyite in a Tsarist palace. But my main reason for soaking up this blissful atmosphere and listening to the beautiful organ melodies swirling around the vast interior has nothing to do with worship or demented political pondering. I just needed an outlet for how I'm feeling. Because if this is a 'high' church, I'm the highest person here.

When I assumed this position a moment ago, grinning like the Cheshire Cat, it felt less like sitting down and more like melting into the furniture. I'm giving the women seated around me marks out of 10, discovering few below eight.

It takes all my resolve to stifle a fit of the giggles when I realise my T-shirt still reeks of the joint I finished earlier, enough to draw several knowing looks. But no more than that. I'm sure there are no *thou shalt nots* in their prized book about hydroponically-produced psychoactive drugs. Although the passages about feeding 5,000 with seven loaves of bread and a few small fish, not to mention the parting of seas, must have been scribed by someone out their face.

This obsession with religion began when I bumped into the daughter of one of Mum's friends. Rosie lived in our street and was part of the gang when we played outside as kids. Now aged 24 and married, she enthused about St Mary's. Like myself, she was christened into the Kirk but was drawn to the more flamboyant Episcopalian service. As a diffident teetotaller she was also attracted to its lively social scene, with diverse clubs run by the high percentage of young adult churchgoers. In my hyperactive condition, I equated this with a potential pool of laid-back single females.

There is a fine line between mainstream religions such as this and the numerous cults which have twisted off on more hedonistic paths. There's a definite hippy vibe with a lot of the females I'm clocking here.

Velvet curtains swish aside. Flanked by subordinates, the priest enters. Lifting his arms, white robes billow. The congregation stands. Many raise their right palms in what appear to be fascist salutes. I realise their pinkies and index fingers are apart, referencing the crucifixion.

A few prayers, some chanting, and a gospel-style hymn later, I'm buzzing with visual, aural, and sensual overload. Satiating my senses with the Holy Spirit, my head is spinning. All the silver crosses capture the sun filtering through the multicoloured windows at the same moment to burn like fluorescent strip lights. Everywhere I look there are gorgeous females with inane smiles, eyes closed, their features betraying how much they have abandoned themselves to the moment.

I feel as if I'm being drawn into something I've never experienced before. Some fantastical dimension. I study ornate tapestries. Awesome stained-glass windows. Flickering candles. I grin at Christ on his cross, towering above us all, features as chiselled as a catwalk model, his dying moments presented as a thing of aesthetic beauty rather than a sordid public execution. In the classic Western supremacist depiction, he is also white-skinned and blue-eyed, like the painting I remember from the room reserved for the Sunday School infants, dripping in irony: an ethnic cross-section of the world's children gazing lovingly at their Aryan Messiah.

But I am enraptured. As the service gets underway again, I feel myself being swept up by the organ music piping through the immense Gothic structure, the otherworldly melodies echoing with the communal voice of hundreds.

When I dip into whatever the priest is rambling about, I hear *I am the resurrection and the light*. He's referencing The Stone Roses. This makes me feel joyous. Overcome with emotion, tears slither down my cheeks. This entire sensory experience is so overwhelming I feel I truly am in the presence of God.

This certainty lasts until I sense the onslaught of the hangover that has been lurking like a mugger. This envelops me with the ferocity of treading on a booby trap. Instead of rupturing limbs, it spears my skull. Behind my eyes, my pulse synchronises with the rhythm of the upbeat hymn everyone else is singing with such verve, accelerating in tempo to leave it far behind.

Paranoia overwhelms euphoria. I grip the cold, varnished wood of the pew in front. I know everyone in the vicinity is aware of my predicament. That heartbeat is thundering now. Pounding in my eardrums. My legs tremble. I feel the sensation of blood seeping as if some invisible vampire is gorging on me. I know I'm about to projectile vomit.

Heaving myself up, I sprint down the aisle, past a sea of bemused faces, focusing on the sunlight bathing the entrance.

Tourists stroll by brandishing cameras and maps. Sparrows chirrup from the trees. The one thing out of the ordinary is lurking just outside the doorway of this late 19th-century cathedral. Leaning into the Victorian brickwork, I fight the urge to throw my guts up like a scene from *The Exorcist*, inhaling the cool air as if my lips are puckered around a roach.

Nausea subsides. I'm already thinking of a million things to do next.

3

Doctor Imposter

October 1987

Peering into the street I see the car has gone. In the dining room, there's a letter on the table. My parents will be explaining why they've left. After the weeks of Hell I've been putting them through, they've decided to abandon me. Some essentials packed. Slipping away before I showed face.

Lifting the note I pace over to the window. Wary of curtains shifting. Whenever I gaze outside, I'm aware of neighbours trying to catch a glimpse of the weirdo in their street.

Hands trembling, I open it. Instead of Mum's handwriting, it's typewritten, the headed paper addressed 'Craiglockhart Surgery.' Signed by Dr McCabe.

After my last appointment, I revealed the truth about McCabe to my parents. He's an imposter. Runs with the Rangers casuals. The Inter City Firm. A mob who've filched their name from West Ham United's hooligans, and their club's East Belfast prejudices.

I saw through those fake certificates pinned to the wall. McCabe has cameras hidden in his surgery. He might issue a modicum of medical advice. But his chief motivations are football violence. Bigotry. Blackmail.

Mum has underlined something in red pen. *Bipolar Disorder*. Reminds me of those cryptic clues from *The Scotsman* crossword they pore over. After consulting the dictionary which also sits on the table, Mum has written on the back of the letter:

Bipolar. Now used to describe manic depression. Manic and/ or depressive episodes. Mental condition. Alternating periods of elation and depression. Mood changes/cycles can happen weekly, monthly, much further apart?

The front door opens. I hear them heaving shopping bags inside. This does nothing to appease my paranoia. They're on the *verge* of deserting me. Maybe not today. Soon. After folding the letter away, I retreat to my bedroom.

When did this *bipolar* start? What started it? Was it one event? Or a combination of them, shunting into each other like a motorway pileup. If so, what triggered that first vehicle to slam on its brakes in the fog? My fertile imagination unspools 11 years to the beginning of my teens. When a summer afternoon transformed into the worst day of my life.

4

The Helper

June 1976

Andy and I are gazing into the burn. I'm sniggering at the way the current makes our faces melt. But not just cause of that. My forced giggles are filling the awkward silences.

Andy's a friend. A schoolfriend. *Not* a mate. Kenny's my best mate. I wish he was here. He's much louder than me. Cheeky. Always prises me out of my shell. Bouncing off me. Giving me the confidence to give as good as I get. Kenny doesn't do silences. He'd be ripping the piss out of us. *Especially* Andy.

Kenny's old man's a prison officer. It's been less than a year since he was transferred to Saughton from Barlinnie. He stands out like a sore thumb at Tynecastle with the Celtic hoops he was told he couldn't wear at PE. And his intimidating, sweary Glasgow accent. He gained respect amongst the bullies by winning a square-go with another second year. Burst his nose in the swing park next to the Westfield flats. All over in under a minute. So he's a useful playground ally where you get picked on if you're shy and told to stop hogging the conversation. *Hate* that.

I like hanging out with Kenny when there are girls around. It's fun listening to them banter. When he flirts with lassies, I'm almost inspired to join in. When he isn't around, I just retreat into shyness. He wouldn't be seen dead at anything as uncool as *this*. A Presbyterian Sunday school picnic.

Andy isn't popular, mostly down to an incident last year. He was too shy to ask our Maths teacher, Mrs Corney to go to the toilet. Whispers spread through the class. He was sitting in a pool of his piss. Kenny's nicknames, never said to his face, are to do with his football team. Pape. Fenian. Bead-rattler. All that moronic nonsense. Andy is just Pissy.

Sometimes he invites me into his house on the way back from school. We drink coffee after coffee until I'm twitching like a bird in a cage. He plays his big brother's albums. Wishbone Ash. The Eagles. Sutherland Brothers and Quiver. They're *awful*.

Against this backdrop of horrible music played by musicians who, like his brother, have shoulder-length manes and wear *massive* flares, Andy and I have dumb conversations about dating girls in our class. There's more chance of Ian Paisley leaving his wife for Mother Theresa. Or as Kenny would say: *Only way youse pair are winching is if youse snaffle some chloroform from the fucking chemistry lab.*

Another warped face appears. When I about turn, I recognise the church guy who travelled with Andy and me in the back of a transit van, stacked high with fold-up tables. During the half-hour journey, we perched on picnic chairs. Now I see how tall he is. Kenny would have dropped his voice to approximate Lurch from *The Addams Family* and said, *you rang?*

He murmurs something about Reverend MacDonald saying there's a tap inside an outhouse. Would I like to fill an urn for making tea? He hands me one. Tells Andy he's to help set up picnic tables.

I shrug. I didn't even volunteer to come to this picnic. Andy phoned first thing this morning. Catching me unawares. Too sluggish to come up with an excuse. He sometimes phones on Saturdays to cajole me into playing cricket at Meggetland. I enjoy cricket. Sometimes you can't be arsed. I know it's him. If my folks are out and my wee sister, Anne's out, the phone keeps ringing until I have to haul myself out of bed and answer. Just to stop the irritating noise.

Why didn't I ignore him? I wouldn't be here, right now, feeling so awkward. Hours of this baking hot afternoon still yawning before me. This isn't even my Sunday school. Andy goes to Cairns Memorial Church in Gorgie. I attend North Merchiston in Shandon. I don't know anyone else here, although I recognised Reverend MacDonald. He's also our school Minister. Mum suggested I might make new friends.

Andy scuffs back towards the picnic site. Glancing at the man, shyness envelops me like a cloak. Made worse cause he never bothered introducing himself when we clambered inside to join him in the van. Andy never did. There was no conversation, though the three of us chuckled each time we went over a bump and got jostled, like the *Star Trek* bridge when the *Enterprise* comes under fire.

We stroll along a gravel path through the trees, around the back of the mansion. I consider asking him if he knows anything about this place. Andy told me it's called Carberry Tower. Instead, I stare at my footfall. My scuffed baseball boots.

I peer sideways. He's middle-aged. Hair shaved around the sides, Brylcream through the top. Shining in the sunlight. This makes him seem out of place in 1976. I could picture him rushing towards a Spitfire. Except he'd struggle to fit inside. Maybe a Lancaster.

I switch my attention to the mansion. Some connection with Mary, Queen of Scots? We did a project on her at primary. Coach trips to different castles. There might have been a battle near here?

The only time he speaks is to announce a game we can play. He'll walk me the rest of the way. When I just gawk, he halts. Asks me to pass him my urn. Holding both urns by their handles, he invites me to face him, stand on his feet, and wrap my arms around him. He indicates his shoes, assuring me he can take my weight. My embarrassment quashes any notion to question this weird development. Blood rushing to my cheeks, I stand on his shiny brown brogues. Clasp his midriff.

He starts trudging along the path, forcing me to tighten my grip to balance. Clenching the urns, he rests his left palm on my shoulder to keep me steady as we stomp along. Getting into a rhythm. My baseball boots are gripping, but he grasps my backside now and again. To make sure I don't stumble. That's what I tell myself.

Being propelled in this bizarre way is sort of adventurous. Except. Each time his hand makes contact to counter the momentum, he gives a squeeze. Looking up, I notice that oily head. I struggle to think of something to say about his greasy hairstyle. To distract him from his pinching fingers. *Anything*. As we bounce along, I hear a mouse-like rustling in the undergrowth. A wren chatters.

I flashback to a holiday in St Abbs. I was eight. Bird spotting with Dad in Berwickshire woodland we came across a wren, motionless in the grass. Peering into the trees I searched for the magpie or owl that had left it for dead. But the branches were deserted. Lifting it, I carried it to the Cortina, clutched it all the way back to our holiday home. Felt its warmth and tiny heartbeat. In the kitchen, I placed it inside a cardboard box in a nest of scrunched up newspapers. Tried feeding it milk. I think of my attempt to fix that wee creature. To bring it back to life. And how upset I was when I knew it had died. I feel that way now. About to burst into tears. I know something is so wrong.

Now he's kneading my bum like dough. He begins whistling. I recognise the melody he is mangling. Brotherhood of Man, the recent Eurovision winners. *Save all your kisses for me.*

We arrive at the outhouse. Shoving the door open he pushes me inside. Forces the door shut. I feel as if we are the last two people on Earth. Every sound becomes magnified. The breeze sends branches scraping against the grimy panes. Skeletal fingers. Tears of moisture run down the glass. A fat spider lurks in its web, surrounded by wasp husks.

The helper's nostrils make a tiny hiss when he breathes out. It sounds funny. I want to tell him it sounds funny. He steers me towards the tap. Holds out the first urn. I grasp this, take its weight. He switches on the tap. I study his hands. The fingernails are long but clean. When the urn is full, he reaches over, prises the handle from my grip, places it to the side.

Turning me around, he throws an arm around my shoulder. Draws me closer. I feel stiffness at his crotch and gasp.

His left hand ruffles my hair. He kisses the top of my head, the way the only person has ever done is Mum. As he keeps massaging my backside, I screw my eyes but open them straight away.

I shudder when he slips his fingers down the gap between my jeans and underpants. Working their way beyond the elastic, they dig until they are inside, between denim and cotton. Begin a rough caressing. Like stroking a pet dog. I want to ask if he's got a pet dog. A mammal he feeds and walks and treats with love and kindness and will be upset about when it dies. He continues this motion while gripping my shoulders with his free hand. He stares. Expressionless. He almost looks as if what he is doing bores him. His breathing betrays a slight emotion. Pinpricks of sweat glisten beneath that lank hair.

I start when he plucks my cardigan's zip, drawing it down. He glances at my Hibs top, the one I was going to reveal to everyone at this Gorgie Sunday school picnic later. He tuts.

The only sound he has made since securing the door. Capturing a solitary sunbeam filtering through the grime, its emerald green has never looked so beautiful. This is why tears come as he gropes at the material, finding my left nipple. Pinching.

As this horror unfolds, I close my welling eyes. Think of the last game at Easter Road. A 2-0 win over Celtic on a Wednesday night three months ago. Alex McGhee scored the first. I picture myself in the Cowshed, the moment Lindsay Muir was hacked down to give us the penalty which Ally MacLeod converted, ending Celtic's championship dreams. The joy of ribbing Kenny the next day.

My mind swirls further. Clutching at the outside world. I visualise what my family will be doing. Sitting around the table. Having lunch. Radio 2 in the background. Earlier I heard The Wurzels, 'Combine Harvester,' then Thin Lizzy's new single, 'The Boys Are Back in Town.'

A mental lifeline. I clutch at the image of Phil Lynott on *Top of the Pops*. Glowering into the camera. Clenching his leather-gloved fist. *If the boys wanna fight you better let 'em.* I bunch my fist. How would a 13-year-old Phil Lynott have reacted to this? Punched the guy's throat. Left him coughing his blood onto the floor, then gone on to write a song about it which would've ended up on *Jailbreak*.

I'm drawn to a strand of his fringe dangling over his face. Quivering with every loathsome movement. That hairstyle. Who looks like that in 1976? No one. Except. Except for a photograph from an article in a Sunday magazine Mum was reading once. An emotionless face to mask sheer evil. Ian

Brady. A sick tribute? The windows are so grubby we're invisible to the outside world. When he's satisfied his urges, no one would see his hands abandoning my groin, closing around my neck. This notion impales me with such terror I have to remember to breathe again.

He burls me round to face the tap. Now his hand makes its way down the front of my jeans. It doesn't feel like a hand at all. As I clock the spider probing towards a wriggling greenfly, this is what I imagine in this claustrophobic mugginess: a monstrous tropical spider creeping towards its prey. This thing starts toying with my balls.

His breath is warm against the back of my neck. The spider legs persist. Clawing. In the shaft of light working its way through a crack in the murky glass, a shadow casts against the ground. His other arm. Jerking. This flickering silhouette is getting faster and with this urgency his fingers are tightening around my cock, making me flinch, tears coursing down my face. His breathing gets harsher. He whispers into my right ear. Something about beautiful eyelashes. I sense everything, his arm, his remorseless grip, his hot, shallow breaths, rushing towards a terrible climax, the worst thing I could ever have imagined in my life.

Lifting the urn, I pour it over myself. He steps back. Water splatters his jacket. Slops onto the floor. We both stare at the puddle. The way it shimmers. Curls around his shoes.

I turn towards the door. Prising it open, I blink at the fierce sunshine. A coal tit flits through the trees. Tomorrow my family will visit the Botanics and I'll hold my palm out, clutching peanuts, feeding coal tits, blue tits, robins, chaffinches. Feeling a pang of delight as each lands and pecks. That's what I focus on.

I hear the tap. Slamming the outhouse door, he shuts away what he's just done. Passes my urn. As we head back, side by side this time, he chats about the feast awaiting us. Erasing the previous minutes. He asks where I live.

Sighthill, I mutter. My outright lie is angelic compared to his perversions. If there is someone up there watching everything, I pray this guy gets punished in *this* life. I doubt I was his first. Or his last. He marches ahead, water sloshing. I want to scream, *you fucking bloody bastard* and stick up the vickies like I did right into a bully's face at Middleton school camp two years ago.

I gaze into a rhododendron bush. A beautiful pink explosion mocking my despair. Inside its foliage, a hedge sparrow trills its sweet melody. Although I'm numbed, I know it could've been so much worse. He didn't rape me. Didn't force me to suck him.

On the lawn beyond, a game of rounders is underway. I spy Andy lunging at the ball. Sending it high. There are shouts of encouragement at the fielders. Reverend MacDonald seizes the ball from the air, provoking a huge cheer.

I stay where I am. Glaring at Andy. Was there something in his expression as he watched me being led away? Something beyond mere relief at not being pressganged into a chore? Something deeper? The more I dwell on this, the greater the gut feeling.

Andy must be aware of gossip in their church? Why didn't he share any suspicions? If not after the van journey, then back at the burn? Did he watch me being led away with relief, glad it wasn't him? Has it been him before? Is this why Andy invited me along, to deflect any ominous attention?

If Kenny was here, he would've told the nonce to fuck off and fill the urns himself. That's what mates do. Not Pissy. Never in a million years. He was too terrified to ask permission to go to the toilet, never mind warn me about this dangerous man.

Maybe I'm being paranoid. Maybe the helper has just never been interested in Andy. But I find that hard to believe. At my scout troop, the 58th Gorgie, the older scouts warn you which leaders to avoid. Especially one nicknamed 'Igor.' *Igor leave my fucking balls alone*, they chant, to the same tune as *you're gonna get your fucking heads kicked in*. Amongst ourselves. This is how kids deal with sex pests like Igor. Or this creep. Or the men who flash at my wee sister and her pals when they're playing in Harrison Park. They're not reported to anyone. Just ridiculed. Behind their backs.

Surely the helper receives the same treatment? Maybe he's more than just a helper. Maybe he's a church officer. A deacon. Maybe the Minister and all the other adults at the Cairns Memorial Church have decided to turn a blind eye. Or try and deflect the blame. I can imagine. *Some teenage boys will say anything to get attention. A lot of them live in a fantasy world at that age, don't they? Especially the quiet ones.*

I can make out the burn. Maybe 15 minutes have elapsed. In these 900 seconds, I feel my life has changed forever.

5

Sniffing Royalty

September 1986

Squinting over *The Scotsman*, Dad tells me I look like a half-shut knife. He mentions the bags under my eyes, then watches my shaking hands struggling to lift my teacup. Muttering about a 20-minute catnap on my bus journey to work, I skim his paper.

Repercussions from last month's Commonwealth Games. Thirty-two out of 59 nations boycotted the competition over Thatcher's refusal to boycott sport in apartheid South Africa. This has left Edinburgh millions in the red.

The *Norsea*, the largest Clyde-built passenger vessel since the *QE2*, was launched by the Queen Mother.

Realising I'm running late, I snatch a slice of toast. From the scullery, Mum asks what time I'm finishing. I reply, when the bank staff say we can.

Seizing a jacket, and munching toast, I bound downstairs. A few steps up the street I turn, waving to my folks at the front room window. Once they're out of sight, I delve into a pocket. Light a Marlboro.

Dad was a smoker at my age. Graduating to occasional cigars in later life, giving up when he retired five years ago. Mum has never smoked, not so much as a draw. An achievement for someone whose teenage years occurred at a time when the majority of adults smoked.

I still feel self-conscious about smoking in front of them. They discovered my vice during a holiday to St Abbs. 1980. Wearing a Siouxsie and the Banshees *Join Hands* T-shirt, I was blowing warped smoke rings outside my mate Richard's caravan when they strolled by. Nothing was said. They just smiled. Waved. I knew they were politely masking their disappointment, which seemed so much worse than an angry reaction.

Whenever Mum empties the ashtray in my bedroom she says it reminds her of Craigentinny. Although Grandad worked in the North British Rubber Mill at Fountainbridge, spending hours in an atmosphere of chemical fumes, he chain-smoked.

The other day, Mum told one of Grandad's stories, about the Queen Mother visiting the factory in 1960. Elizabeth's expensive perfume lingered for days afterwards, signposting the route the royal entourage followed while being escorted around the shop floor. This lingered in a lift, so men would pop inside to sniff her scent, before resuming churning out rubber items as the workforce had been doing for decades.

Including millions of boots for the uniformed men and women fighting and dying for Elizabeth and King George VI two decades before.

I could picture him amongst his workmates, lighting the next fag from the previous one on their breaks. My memories are of a frail man in his 70s in the Northern General, lungs ravaged with emphysema, struggling to whisper to everyone clustered around his bed. His life reduced to these four walls he'd never be leaving. Every so often a nurse would place a plastic mask over his face. A faint smile would crease his lips as he sucked the oxygen, as if he was remembering the Queen Mother's sweet aroma.

When the number 33 pulls up, memories of Grandad fade. Flicking away the dowt, I check the time. At the other end, if I sprint from the bus stop, against the tantalizing scents from the Burton's Biscuits factory, I should reach the bank building by nine.

Trudging upstairs to the back seats, I close my leaden eyelids. Drift into a fitful slumber.

*

This job is characterised by lengthy periods of boredom, interspersed with bursts of activity. While awaiting the next batch of forms for processing, my co-workers and I slouch over tables, chatting, telling jokes, poring over the papers from the headlines to the sport, and back again. I'm struggling to read *Moon* by James Herbert while my fatigued eyesight keeps transforming the text into hieroglyphics.

A voice carries from a couple of tables away. Frankie's sing-along West of Scotland accent is relaying a *Daily Record* story about Pinochet's motorcade being ambushed.

Someone asks who the fuck's Pinochet? A wine producer? Was it some Mafia hit?

Chilean dictator. Not heard of him? Fucksake. His military coup deposed Allende?

And how the fuck are we supposed to know who Allende is? Sounds like someone who played along Souness at Sampdoria.

Allende? Souness? Good guy. Prick. Naw, Charlie. Allende was Chile's democratically elected president. Toppled by the army. With CIA help. Obviously.

Francis Kelly's history lesson of the day.

Listen, Charlie. He was best buds with Maggie Thatcher, milk snatcher. Five of his bodyguards died. But the fascist bastard gets away with a few cuts, fucksake.

Nothing new, Frankie, chips in Iain, my Aussie mate. Big on INXS, less so The Saints. First thing I asked him in the canteen on day one. D'you know there were more than forty plots to bump off Hitler?

Frankie snorts. No wonder the one-bollocked wanker ended up having to do it himself.

The paperback slips through my fingers. Tumbles to the floor. Plucking it up, I head for the toilets, enter a cubicle, and lock the door. Easing onto the seat I fold my arms, head bowed.

A furious thumping wakes me. A Paisley accent. *Fleming? That you in there?*

I blurt out: *Frankie?*

He informs me I've been away from my desk for half an hour, skiving cunt that I am, and he's going to grass me to the man. I chuckle at him pretending to be bothered. Also because his tache and unruly curls always remind me of Bobby Ball, if the Oldham-born comic was a St Mirren season ticket-holder.

Rock on, Frankie, I tell him, promising to rejoin the company in a minute.

The outside door creaks open and shut. When I shuffle back to my seat the spontaneous applause my re-appearance instigates from my colleagues draws the attention of the bank supervisor, Veronica. An attractive woman in her early 20s, her sour expression seems tattooed into her features. She empties crates of forms over the desks.

As Veronica clicks away down the corridor, like many of my colleagues, I track her cascading red hair and the subtle wiggle of her backside until she exits.

Frankie fixes me in his sights and informs me none of us would have a fucking snowball's chance with thon. Gets picked up every day by a boy in a Mazda RX-7 Turbo. Red. Fucking naturally.

I have no idea what that is so I can't form a mental picture. But I can still get a hint of her designer perfume.

6

Burnout

Mum is back from shopping with her friend Irene and is passing on news about her daughter. Janice is 20, studying accounting at Napier. Mum tells me Janice was taken ill and had to leave her digs and move home to North Berwick. When I ask what was up with her, Mum pauses, then tells me, a nervous breakdown.

Nervous breakdown? Mum's hesitancy about revealing Janice's condition is countered by my scoffing. For this to be used as a reason for dropping out of her studies just sounds like a convenient excuse.

I picture Janice in a doctor's waiting room, surrounded by pensioners shuffling in for angina pills, pregnant women: people with actual medical conditions. I also visualise a war movie: a GI cowering under Japanese gunfire and shrieking for his mother, John Wayne reacting with a robust slap.

Demanding he pulls himself together. Stops disgracing the Stars and Stripes.

Mum frowns at my lack of empathy and describes what must have been a difficult conversation for Irene in the upstairs café at Frasers. Everything was getting on top of Janice. Too many late nights studying. The pressure of all the coursework. Cramming for exams.

Shrugging, I state accountancy is surely just glorified arithmetic. If Janice worked in air traffic control, I could understand *nervous exhaustion*.

Mum insists not being able to cope is down to individuals. Sometimes it's their chemical make-up, their metabolism, that defines if they fall ill. Janice just got to the point where she couldn't face anything. Just getting out of bed became an ordeal.

I laugh at that one. Welcome to most people's world, I comment, adding Janice might benefit from a good shake rather than whatever medication her GP prescribed. A large tumbler of sherry always provided the perfect antidote to stress the morning before any of my Napier exams.

Mum insists Janice is almost teetotal. Probably drinks less over one term than I put away on a night out. This observation instils a sense of pride rather than admonishment. In Scotland, beer bellies are a badge of honour. And The Duke, in or out of character, knew how to deal with *nervous breakdowns*.

7

Mystery Girls

May 1987

Sunday nights in Buster Brown's are even busier than Saturdays, always rammed with hairdressers who get the Monday off. There's a cool vibe. Some might say elitist.

Rather than inflicting cheesy Top 20 dance music on the clientele, the DJs spin the latest Chicago House imports. Interspersed with classic soul. Funk. Hip-hop. Anyone spotted dancing around handbags to 'Love Can't Turn Around,' by Farley Jackmaster Funk is liable to be ejected by the bouncers.

Popular enough for the queue to snake towards Waverley Bridge, it never begins filling up until after midnight. This means when I head along with Alex, Grum, and the final member of our regular quartet, Dougie to take advantage of the early Happy Hour, we have the place to ourselves.

Each of us buys a double round. By the time punters start trickling in after other pubs have closed we're already many drinks into the improbable collection of 32 pints, bottles and nips clustered around a circular table by the empty dancefloor.

But because this is a 'happening' club rather than what would have been referred to as a disco earlier in the 1980s, it also attracts coachloads from other towns and cities. You might even catch Graeme Souness or Ally McCoist at the bar, corralled by minders, Sol-sipping sycophants hanging on their every word. Regulars include local heroes, Mickey Weir, Gary MacKay, and Jimmy Sandison, getting loaded with mates they'd been at school with.

Gary was at Tynecastle High, two years below me, a mate of one of my best buddies at work, Splodge. His Hearts team-mate, John Robertson married a Shandon girl last year, Tracey, the year below Anne. Her big brother Stuart was in my patrol at Scouts. Edinburgh can be a village.

*

Thinking of last night, I muse that office temps are so much further down the singleton food chain than Scotland's professional footballers. But my hazy recollections are hampered by a remorseless headache.

I'm trying to remember the name of a gorgeous redhead I was dancing with. Although dancing is a generous description of shambolic movements fuelled by double-figure Red Stripes, OVD Rum and Crabbie's Green Ginger chasers, augmented by spliffs shared in the area furthest from the radar of any bouncers, what my mates and I refer to as 'smoker's corner' behind the DJ booth. The phone number she scrawled onto my Marlboro packet referred to a hair salon – in Dunfermline? – but it's long been smudged, the numbers indecipherable.

Less than six hours after my last drink, my gaze returns to the forms. British Airways is being privatised, the Thatcher government's latest initiative to eviscerate a public service by offering cash incentives to hundreds of thousands of budding capitalists across the UK. Along with the selling off of council houses and siphoning the profits from North Sea oil into the London Stock Exchange rather than investing it into a fund for the future, her ideology is transforming the face of Britain, smashing its industrial heartland to rubble with a clinical efficiency Hermann Göring could only have dreamt about.

We temporary clerks are but cogs in this relentless erosion of the public sector, having been hired by the Royal Bank of Scotland for several months of soul-destroying processing of share applications.

The task at hand is simple enough for primates to make a fist of it after basic training. We send letters to customers informing them how much of their requested share application they are being allocated. The names and addresses have to be handwritten, the details transposed from computer printouts. As well as having to cope with a splitting headache and intermittent spells of nausea, I'm wrestling with post-alcoholic quivers that transform much of my address writing into a cardiograph's squiggles. Pacing along the desks doing spot checks, Veronica insists I print particular addresses again.

Each time reminding the entire floor how wasteful it is to bin useless forms.

The one favourable aspect of this work is it's well remunerated. Because I was a Napier student up until I graduated in the summer I'm on a low tax threshold. This is offset by the drudgery. Clocking-off can be anytime between six and nine. This particular evening the senior bank supervisor tells us to down pens at five past nine.

*

I jog up to the Calder Road and sprint for a 22, jumping off at the Foot of the Walk, the interminable journey lasting long enough to smoke three tabs.

Pacing through the deserted Kirkgate, I skulk beneath the Linksview towerblock, heading for Queen Charlotte Street. Casting a wary eye on a posse of youths tearing past on bikes, whooping like a Sioux raiding party in a Hollywood movie, I wonder if they're outriders for the Young Leith Team. Tension. Excitement. Sets the mood for the impending activity.

8

Leith Band Agnes

Climbing the dilapidated building's rickety staircase, a cacophony assails my senses. I pick out Fini Tribe's 'De Testimony,' with its anthemic chimes and jerking bassline. They did a Peel session two years back. They've since ditched guitars and got a hold of a sampler. Now they'd ram the Buster's dancefloor if the DJs could see beyond US house imports.

Barging into our practice room, the guys are involved in an ear-shredding jam. Tom, face contorted, blowing into his clarinet, a snake charmer surrounded by writhing cobras. Kenny, his fingers slapping then sliding along the fretboard, bass jerking in time with the rhythm. Jack forsaking his trademark beaters for the sticks necessary to maintain a pulverising beat.

I pace over to my Orange amp and plug in the guitar I left at Tom's Leith Walk flat the previous weekend, a Fender Strat stencilled with LEITH BAND AGNES. This is our band's pseudonym – the actual name is Little Big Dig. But one of our songs was released on a compilation album earlier this year, *Wide Open*, under that nom-de-plume. The term 'song' is also a stretch as it was an improvised piece recorded in one take, entitled 'Dr Buck Ruxton,' its subject a 1930s serial killer, one of the first cases to be solved by forensic evidence. It was also wonderfully crooned by Tom's mother.

Awaiting me are purple tins of Tennent's Super. Flipping one open, the first mouthfuls are treacherous, but working up to several greedy slugs achieves a reassuring numbness. This sense of relaxation prompts me to launch an angular guitar line over Kenny's riff once I've sussed his root notes. Bb, E, and A.

I nudge the volume higher. I spend my weekends dancing ineptly to soul and house. Dig produce far more visceral post-rock. Dipping into the aural escapism of Can.

The piece finds its natural conclusion, my final crashing chord fading into reverb. Tom strides over to his tape recorder, hits the 'stop' button. I stumble as I bend down to fiddle with my effects pedals. Easing the overdrive down a notch, I play a few chords with a less abrasive setting. Kenny launches into a lugubrious bassline with a quirky, jazzy undertone.

I set off on some jagged lead improvisation, not a million miles away from something Bruce Gilbert might've done on Wire's *154*. Tom adds a plaintive keyboard refrain while Jack kicks into a shuffling rhythm using his beaters.

As Tom begins picking out a repetitive melody, he catches my eye and nods to the recorder. Pausing on a D minor bar-chord, I step over. Press 'play/record.'

From its dulcet overture, this next jam builds into an even more menacing piece. At one point Tom is stabbing at the keyboard while I'm plucking strings way up the fretboard, then pressing my guitar into the amp to submerge any lingering melody beneath a squall of feedback. The bass pummels, Kenny playing chords while Jack switches to sticks and begins thrashing the cymbals.

At synchronised intervals, the sonic wall dips into a gorgeous key change. The 8.4% lager already working its magic on my senses, this divergence puts me in mind of a chink of sunlight during a storm. The hiatus persists for several bars before the music gains momentum, clawing towards new heights. Or sinking into murkier depths.

Like so many twentysomething rock musicians devoted to their art, I harbour delusions that what we are doing will lead to my escape from the mundane crap that approximates my profession. I'm adamant any serious record producer hearing our demos will see pound signs. After all the twee jangly-guitar pop polluting the post-punk scene like Bible Belt summer campfire singalongs, our mood pieces will inject long overdue shades of twisted darkness.

The track winds down until Jack concludes with swirling crashes on the cymbals that remind me of storm clouds receding. As he adjusts the position of his kit, his beam reflects what we are all thinking: what we have just recorded was, as Tom always describes these events, 'a happening.' Nothing needs articulating. Each of us played an integral role in creating this fantastic piece of music: a cocktail of Can, The Fall, Wire, and The Residents that snatched elements of those bands to produce a unique musical cocktail.

Tom will take the cassette home and analyse it over the next few days, suggesting a more formalised structure for the ragged loose ends. Not to jam a square into a circle by imposing a straightjacket template of verse, chorus, break, and so on. To haul it back from being a one-off improvisation into something we can imitate in future, refining the key changes and fine-tuning the solos. Most importantly, he'll incorporate his idiosyncratic lyrics.

Tom's prose is far removed from the quasi-political slogan-eering that inspired my songwriting in the days of my first band, 4 Minute Warning. They're closer to poetry than anything I could muster.

I've always been drawn to The Fall vocalist Mark E Smith's ability to apply what seem like random snatches from a stream of consciousness to paint abstract but potent images. One that springs to mind after watching The Fall's *Perverted By Language* video in the small hours of this morning: *Winston Churchill had a speech imp-p-p-pediment, and look what he did, he razed half of London*. My attempts to follow suit come across as half-baked impersonations of the Mancunian word-smith. So I'm content to leave the lyrics in Tom's far more capable hands.

He shares Smith's effortless ability to conjure mental pictures, from an angle unique to Central Scotland rather than

Salford. Tom's observations attest to the records cramming the shelves of his flat: Ivor Cutler, Iggy Pop, Captain Beefheart, Tom Waits.

An example: *How's that for a middle-shed, a carving knife, in the head?* Or my favourite, from a magnificent piece containing the guitar solo I'm proudest of, 'Big Fire at the Stampworks.' Surreally, this references a custody battle involving Hitler and Mussolini, climaxing as a paean to Dudley D Watkins, genius illustrator of The Broons. Celebrating how his mesmerising cartoons depict a timeless working-class Scottish culture and make hangovers bearable: *Comfort me, comfort me, Dud-dud-Dudley D.*

There are shedloads of irony. 'Leith Walk Limbo,' a song from our set when we had a residency in La Sorbonne in 1985, was inspired by a Tom Waits gig just after he released his album *Rain Dogs*. The concert was a sell-out, but Tom and flatmate Jack left it too late to get tickets. They happened to be passing the Playhouse just as the man himself was exiting after sound-checking. Tom from Ayr, a massive fan of Tom from California, spent 15 minutes engaging in starstruck chat, the latter adding their names to his guest list.

They were so overawed by this unforeseen turn of events they spent the rest of the afternoon fuelling themselves with Tennent's Super. Arriving at the venue they were refused admittance. A distraught Tom told me the bouncer took one look at them and said, *guest list my arse, pair of youse're fucking Owen Archdeacon.*

The port of Leith's main thoroughfare also featured during an abortive reworking of a Simon & Garfunkel classic, re-titled: 'The Only Living Boy in Leith Walk.' Another cover we've tampered with is 'Stolen Kisses,' by Psychic TV, formed by Throbbing Gristle vocalist/visual artist Genesis P-Orridge and Alternative TV's founding guitarist Alex Fergusson. Despite the former's avante-garde songwriting legacy, it's a jangly pop song.

Our song titles can also be an education. One we may well conclude the practice with tonight: 'Paleoweltschmerz.' I'd never heard of this before Tom sprung it on us. It's the theory that the reason for the dinosaur extinction wasn't the fallout from an ancient meteor strike so devastating it disrupted the earth's climate. It was boredom.

Tom sparks a roll-up, enough left for a couple of game draws, grinds it out. I spot a rough set-list he has been jotting down in preparation for our next gig, later this month at The Jailhouse. A double-header with our regular co-performers, Teenage Dog Orgy – a 'supergroup' consisting of Martin, Goodbye Mr Mackenzie's vocalist/guitarist, Paul, singer with Kitsch and the Night Set, and Billy and Gordon, bassist and drummer from The Calloways.

We played there in the summer of 1985, performing twice, on a Saturday afternoon, then again at night. The earlier set consisted of actual songs, some of the ones we were earmarking for our debut album. 'Janie.' 'Humour and the Human Being.' 'The Beautiful Suit.' 'Do the Dirty.' 'Mouseface.' 'Big Fire at the Stampworks.' 'Sleep is Good.' All poppy post-punk gems.

The evening material consisted of one-off songs, including a cover of Hank Williams' 'Your Cheatin' Heart' and a catchy original, 'Sons of the Desert,' our tribute to history's greatest comic act, Laurel and Hardy. We jammed these perched on bar stools, wearing white shirts and bow ties.

As the night wore on and drink was taken, we began improvising tracks, incorporating samples from a large reel-to-reel recorder. There was a doom-laden instrumental we'd laid the backing track for, 'Tay Bridge Disaster.' Another, inexplicably named 'Keemie the Schemie,' set off on a weirdly plaintive riff I'd concocted, reminiscent of some Moroccan jazz club, but driven by Kenny's dense, Jay Wobblesque bassline. The backing tape was a looped recording from Coronation Street, Kevin Webster coming on to his church-going girlfriend Michelle but getting the brush off.

We closed with a drawn-out wall of noise entitled 'Macbeth Theme.' Both sets were taped; the earlier one ending in rapt applause and encores of older songs, 'You are my Sweetie Shop' and 'Hard on Heart,' the latter to awkward silence, broken by clinking classes and conversations around the horseshoe bar.

For our triumphant return, I'll have to invent a dental emergency to enable me to escape work. This time, the core of the set will be new songs, although a couple have survived from the ill-fated Arran session under the ever-wishful heading of encores.

In October 1985 we embarked on the ferry from Ardrossan, laden with overnight bags and musical equipment. Quaffing Guinness while standing at the prow, chortling as the ship ploughed through the towering swell, any notion of seasickness was countered by excitement at the weekend ahead.

We were booked into an isolated cottage owned by a guy Tom knew from Ayr, Malcolm, who ran a recording studio from a spare room. We would lay down nine songs for the debut album we intended releasing in cassette format. Malcolm's speciality was analogue equipment, including a reel-to-reel tape recorder. This bulky machine's 2-inch reel-to-reel tapes would create the demos, before these were copied to 0.15-inch cassettes, channelling the original audio signal intact. This would result in high-fidelity quality recordings, superior to cassette-to-cassette copies and equal to vinyl reproduction.

Jack had already completed the artwork to be replicated for the handouts to accompany each numbered cassette. Once we had the pristine, penultimate version, our backing singer, Donna, would add her harmonies. The cake's glorious icing.

Winding down after our first day's creativity, we finished the carryout we bought earlier, continued drinking in Brodrick, finding our way to a hotel, before gatecrashing a local girl's 21st until that function room's bar closed.

Swaying back to our digs, the conversation turned to a snippet of information Malcolm offered with a mischievous glint when handing over the keys to the two caravans outside: our accommodation. This field marked the location of an extensive 11th-century Viking burial ground.

With the wind whistling through telephone lines, this ominous detail gained prominence. Although we had opted to split into two twos for crashing out, Kenny and Jack in one caravan, Tom and myself in the other, Tom now insisted he was going to sleep here on the floor. My intoxication outweighing the notion of murderous Nordic ghosts, I opted for Plan A. Grasping a ring pull containing three cans, I stomped over to the second caravan.

I discovered a threadbare cushion. Lying flat transformed my berth into a waltzer. Recalling Malcolm had stuffed pillows into his studio speakers for sound dampening, I decided to fetch one.

The front door was unlocked in case any of us needed access to the toilet. Creeping along the hall and into the studio, I groped for a light switch. After unsuccessful pawing, I continued inside. My eyes growing more accustomed to the gloom, I spotted a speaker. Stretching towards it, my legs impacted the cable leading to the massive reel-to-reel machine, triggering an almighty crash.

It felt as if I'd bumbled into a booby trap. I gawked at the indistinct hulk of the recording apparatus now face-down on the floor. Heaving it up, I plonked it back into an approximation of its original position, although it was now balancing on a spaghetti-like cluster of wires. But like that Laurel and Hardy scene when Stan emerges from the wreckage of the fishing boat his carelessness has just destroyed, grinning after discovering his horn intact, I secured my pillow and careened out.

In the morning my slumber was interrupted by Tom poking his head inside to inform me Kenny had just left to catch the next ferry.

Why?

Because he was desperate to make it to Tannadice for Hibs away that afternoon.

Why, when we still had four tracks to record?

His answer was curt and knowing. Somehow Malcolm's recorder, the one which set him back a four-figure sum, fell from its shelf during the night, one of the delicate spindles holding the reels snapping. In terms of its ability to record our album, this apparatus was now about as much use as his fucking toaster.

Our ferry journey back to the mainland took place under a denser cloud than the grey skies rolling in from Ireland. My only saving grace was managing to persuade Dad to drive 80 miles to collect us. My inadvertent sabotage had scuppered what was supposed to make up for the debacle the previous year, at the BBC Maida Vale studios.

At the time we were such a 'going places' band we had a manager, Alex. He'd played in a group, Family Von Trapp, Glasgow Art College graduates we got to know when they shared our first practice room in Niddry Street. Also in the band was his girlfriend, Muriel Gray, now a co-presenter on *The Tube*. We once popped into their Elm Row flat to chat about gigs and recordings. Feeling starstruck as Muriel made coffees.

She also stood in for DJs on *BBC Radio 1* and when presenting Richard Skinner's show had been given free rein to book a couple of unknown Scottish bands. This gifted us with a golden opportunity for nationwide exposure. Armed with guitars, keyboards, and bulky carryout bags, Tom, Jack and myself, along with Colin and his partner, Susan, respectively our original bassist and backing vocalist, boarded the night bus to London from Waverley Bridge, convinced this marked the first leg of our journey into fame.

Our BBC engineer was none other than Dale Griffin, former drummer of Mott the Hoople, famous for the glam rock anthem 'All the Young Dudes,' written for them by David Bowie. That connection continued when Mick Ronson, the multi-talented musician from Hull instrumental in Bowie's meteoric rise joined Mott the Hoople in 1974.

The night before our trip to the BBC studios, we stayed in the North London residence of the actor, Graham Crowden. His son, Harry lived in Edinburgh and was a good mate. A long-time fan of each of my bands, he also introduced me to my first serious girlfriend, Louise in 1981.

A regular collaborator with the film director Lindsey Anderson, a leading light of the 1960s New Wave of British Cinema, Graham was mainly a stage actor now. He also popped up in diverse TV roles. Once a prison doctor in *Porridge*, he was approached to become the fourth Dr Who after Jon Pertwee. He turned it down to avoid being typecast.

Not sleeping much in an unfamiliar bed, Graham poured a generous gin and tonic in the morning. Getting a lift to the studios in West Kilburn from Graham's wife, Phyllida, we stopped off to purchase our staple poison: litre bottles of Merrydown Cider, ABV 8.2%.

We were in awe of being added to Griffin's CV, an impressive roster that included Pulp's first professional recording session in 1981, and The Smiths' Peel sessions, broadcast before they'd released any records, tracks that would resurface on their 'Hatful of Hollow' compilation.

The long day began with us launching into the first of our four tracks, charged with excitement, enthusiasm, and strong cider. The obvious difference from running through these songs over months of rehearsals was a prominent wall light flashing red to indicate a take. Providing an adrenaline jolt to focus our attention, each time Colin's bassline was a semitone out, Jack missed a cymbal crash, or my fingers ambushed a chord progression, this beacon cutting out stoked tension.

Progressing to overdubs, I was alone in the studio to add an acoustic guitar overdub to our final track, 'Nothing Much At All.' My arms were trembling as if the fretboard was live. Between the many takes, I kept swigging Merrydown as if I was seeking inspiration from teenage binges in the parkie's shed at Harrison Park.

Getting through the four and a half minute rhythm guitar accompaniment seemed to take as many hours. When Griffin's assistant spoke into my headphones to say the last version sounded champion, it felt like reaching the line after a gruelling cross-country race.

Back by the mixing desk, I eased in between Susan and Jack on the bench opposite a vast deck of switches and flickering dials. I became engrossed by Griffin manipulating the controls, replaying my track, nudging the volume and tone to blend in with my lead guitar line.

Studying his fluid movements, all I could think of was that these digits had once kept the rhythm for Mick Ronson, lead guitarist, enigmatic Spider from Mars. Ronson's first-ever session with Bowie took place in this very studio in 1970 when 14 songs were recorded for a Peel session.

These included six tracks from his psychedelic and folky second album, *Space Oddity*, and a cover of The Velvet Underground's 'I'm Waiting for the Man.'

Ronson was brought into the frame because Bowie and his producer Tony Visconti wanted to move in a bold new direction, ditching wistful folk in favour of loud rock, inspired by The Stooges and Velvets Bowie had listened to during his first visit to America the month before. Ronson's electrifying guitar sound telegraphed this seachange in Bowie's career.

Performing 'Starman' on *Top of The Pops* on July 6th 1972, the day after Mum's 40th birthday, the moment a flame-haired Bowie draped an arm around Ronson, pointing down the camera while singing, *I had to phone someone, so I picked on you,* is often cited as the precise moment he became a superstar.

It was also pivotal for the punk generation, the spark that kindled an obsession with music for the teenaged Robert Smith, Richard Jobson, David Gahan, and Gary Kemp; inspiring a young Stuart Goddard, Susan Ballion and Simon Ritchie's journeys to becoming, respectively, Adam Ant, Siouxsie Sioux, and Sid Vicious; in short, spawning the British punk scene, and by extension, my own musical obsessions.

Ronson's collaboration also propelled the rise of glam rock. Bowie's subsequent albums, *The Rise and Fall of Ziggy*

Stardust and the Spiders From Mars and *Alladin Sane* surfed that wave, Ronson's potent riffs, performed on his vintage Gibson Les Paul, 'Ziggy' integral to this sonic revolution.

I'm always thrilled by vicarious connections. Like Graham's stories at the breakfast table when he recounted drinking sessions with Yul Brynner, Christopher Lee, Richard Harris, and Malcolm McDowell.

During the lengthy mixing process, Griffin's assistant explained the rough edges and bum notes we insisted on re-recording would get smoothed over in the final mix. While he assuaged us, Griffin muttered under his breath, irritated by the amount of cider we were guzzling. He became agitated at our bellowed suggestions in slurred Scottish brogues. The straw that broke the camel's back was a beaker of cider decanting over the carpet tiles next to the bank of equipment responsible for mixing everyone from The Beatles to Led Zeppelin, Bowie to Hendrix, and every John Peel session since 1967, including seven by The Fall.

Heading back out of London, we were consumed with the notion an opportune moment had slipped out of our hands.

Our session was broadcast on 17th July 1984, the night before I turned 22. I listened with Dad, and he took a photo of the large radio/cassette recorder presented to him at his retiral do two years before that he was using to proudly tape it.

Muriel played our catchiest song, 'You are my Sweetie Shop,' featuring Tom's typically quirky chorus, *It's just as well we don't know what's in front of us, love or disease, an iron bar or a bus.* She introduced it by referencing that if there were dance mixes of Frankie Goes to Hollywood, here was a pick and mix.

The other unknown Scottish band she booked for a session came from her hometown. Lloyd Cole and the Commotions. I'm sure they performed their four tracks with consummate professionalism and were impeccably behaved during the mixing. Their debut album, *Rattlesnakes*, sold over 100,000 copies in Britain, reaching number 13 in the charts. I believed the material from the Arran sessions would have produced a memorable album. But we shot ourselves in the foot yet again. Or at least, I did.

When I gulp from my purple tin the *what-ifs* are superseded by *what next?* The doob Jack is handing to me.

*

It is ten to one when I pad into the house. Ears ringing. Eyesight blurred. Burping lager. Mum has left my tea in the microwave. I'm so voracious I burn my tongue.

When I collapse on my bed, the gruelling practice has resulted in tinnitus that now makes me think of the last sound a hapless racing pigeon would hear before being shredded by a jet engine. No matter how fatigued I feel, the noise renders sleep impossible.

So I heave myself up, slink through to Dad's drinks cabinet, and fill a half-pint tumbler with sherry. Creeping back to my bedroom, I squeeze my headphones on, plug in, select *Scared to Dance*, The Skids' masterful debut, dropping the needle onto track four, 'Dossier (Of Fallibility).'

Like the majority of Richard Jobson's lyrics, the subject matter seems obtuse, but so much more complimentary to Stuart Adamson's exploring guitar lines than shouty punk-by-numbers. When I switch off the bedroom light, the glow from the HiFi's display synchronizes with the eerie, minor pentatonic scales, while my swimming vision adds to the hypnotic effect.

Next thing I know the glass is on its side. The album is clicking against the stylus and the headphone cable is wrapped around my neck. Sparrows are chirping in the back green. My body is leaden with exhaustion. The thought of cereal turns my stomach.

I drain the remaining sips of sherry. Just before I sink into the final minutes before the alarm, I notice the note on my bedside cabinet. Mum's fastidious writing: *11.45. Tom phoned. Masterpiece lost forever. You left the pause button on. Idiot!*

9

Can't Stand My Baby

July 1987

Another blackout has erased hours of my life. Memories flicker. Friday night kicked off when we clambered into taxis and fired along to the RBS on the corner of Castle Street to cash our paycheques, heading straight to the Traveller's Tryst, wallets crammed with beer vouchers.

At ten past five, we pounded down the stairs into Styx, assailed by blaring music and the clamour of binge drinkers taking advantage of £1 cocktails.

I started with several glasses of slow comfortable screws up against the wall: a concoction of sloe gin, Amaretto, vodka, Southern Comfort, and orange juice, topped with a cherry. This might as well be called a smash your head against a wall. I followed with three screaming orgasms, the same head-into-wall effect achieved with vodka, Irish cream, and coffee liqueur.

At one point I bumped into Jo Callis, once of The Rezillos. Together with Pete Shelley of Buzzcocks and the O'Neill brothers of The Undertones, these guys were pop punk pioneers. As well as numerous *Top of the Pops* appearances with The Rezillos, including performing their hit single namechecking the show, he wrote most of the Human League's *Dare*.

Starstruck and drunk, I couldn't think of anything impressive to say. Instead, I roared their Fleetwood Mac cover: *Somebody's gonna get their head kicked in tonight!* He beamed at being referenced among the George Street drunkards, most of whom were too young for punk. When our paths crossed again, I changed the record. *I can't stand my baby, it's a real drag, I think I'm going crazy, I'm gonna go radge*!

Later I spotted my mate Alex bending Jo's ear at the bar while waiting to get served. I sidled up beside them. Every time a blonde barmaid flitted by, Alex did that noise at the back of his throat, the weird erotic gargle Roy Orbison does during 'Pretty Woman,' before he returned to his monologue with Jo who was just grinning into his cocktail.

Alex and I were introduced by a mutual friend, Grum, who I knew from school. Although Grum left for a bricklaying apprenticeship and I became an insurance clerk, our friendship was maintained by our overlapping record collections: everything from Alternative TV to Zounds, and countless other lesser-known bands you would hear through John Peel or via the grapevine outside Bruce's – The Wall. The Dark. The Pack. Pseudo Existors. Discharge. Fatal Microbes. XS-Energy. The Fegs. The Licks – singles often released in self-designed sleeves on local presses, a few hundred at a time, going on to become as sought-after by avid collectors as Anglo-Saxon gold.

Alex started working beside Grum and we met in The Diggers one night, hitting it off when he professed his love of anarchic rock 'n' roll – especially The Skids and Big Country.

My best buddies at school were Brian and Kenny. Brian was into ELO. Kenny was a metalhead, viewing punk through a *Daily Mail* prism: a tuneless racket, played too fast, the court jester attire of safety pins and spiky hair anathema to 'birds.' But the small punk contingent at Tynecastle were drawn to the excitement and energy lacking in so many of the drab, lank-haired rock musos churning out showboating solos on *The Old Grey Whistle Test*.

Robert Plant paraphrased Tolkien's ringwraiths and named his pet dog Strider, while his band tossed TVs from five-star hotel windows or rode motorcycles through their lobbies knowing their management would always cover the damage. We were hooked on songs about the modern world and borstal breakouts. Furious outbursts calling out grovelling royalists as morons. Lyrics about unemployment, disaffection, alienation, right-wing thugs. Or in the case of Buzzcocks or The Undertones, nothing more profound than the joy and heartache of teenage love.

Alex was laid off from his last building site contract a few months back. I put in a word with the office staff at the temp agency. His interview was perfunctory, consisting of him flirting with the two lassies firing the questions at him. Now he works beside me, relishing grafting indoors amongst a workforce that is 50% female, and all within the catchment for a Club 18-30 holiday.

*

Dream-like memories of pestering popstars fade into this morning's skull-splitting hangover. Mum chaps the bedroom door, enters with a mug of tea and informs me I'm late for work. Pausing, she waits for any reaction beyond me blinking my bloodshot eyes. I shrug and yawn. She adds I've had around three or four hours sleep, tops. I'm burning my candle at both ends.

Clogged with nicotine, my throat rattles and I suffer a coughing fit. Mum recoils from my breath. Now she castigates my diet, how devouring pizzas in the small hours is the antithesis of a healthy intake, and this has been the case for months. Her other hand is tucked behind her back. Now she waves an envelope in front of me. I thumb it open. My birthday card.

A quarter of a century, she says, although right now you look *forty*-five.

10

The Wolves

As ever, our 30-minute lunch break degenerates into a contest to determine who can sink the most pints and chasers before trudging back upstairs to the office. Since I'm still feeling the after-effects of yesterday's session, and the previous day's, I'm struggling with my third Southern Comfort and lemonade, while my Tennent's lager glass remains untouched. Every so often the barmaid clears empties and gestures towards it while I shake my head, lunging for another sip.

I glower at the TV above the bar, at the plasticine animation for The Firm's 'Star Trekkin.' Ten years on from the high-tide mark of punk 7-inch singles, pop is as garish and disposable as ever but is now propelled by MTV, a 24/7 conveyor belt of addictive earworms. This effervescent backdrop blares from wall-mounted screens like this one across the city centre's trendier bars.

Next in the non-stop chain of aural candy is 'La Bamba' by Los Lobos, the current number 1. A gaggle of drunken voices sing along to the hit that has become the anthem to our binge-ing, its refrain signposting our pub crawls, the first selection from each jukebox, the exultant chorus rising in relation to the alcohol consumed.

I clock Splodge bantering with the barmaid. He can wring humour out of any situation and is on first name terms with most of the clientele in Luckies and The Wheatsheaf. He's more than a good mate. His jovial presence is an asset for everyone sharing his table during the hours of repetitive tasks, although we all accept this also means being on the receiving end of his gibes. Splodge should have a one-man show and is undoubtedly funnier than half the acts who'll tell observa-tional jokes before a paying audience. He can also out-drink any of us.

Last week he discovered a student who started in our team, Gregorio, hails from Buenos Aires. He demanded Gregorio transcribe the song's Spanish lyrics. Splodge can now sing it, word for word, or as the night wears on, noisy slur for slur. Yesterday he popped down here on his own for 'one for the road.' The bar manager, Doug, discovered him passed out in a toilet cubicle at closing time. According to Doug, when he managed to rouse Splodge he roared: *Para bailar la bamba, Para bailar la bamba... Se necesita una poca de gracia... Una poca de gracia!*

The Tex-Mex singalong segueing into Whitney Houston's 'I want to dance with somebody,' becomes the cue for glasses to be drained before the reluctant exodus.

*

For all that the lunchtime session seemed like forcing down medicine, I've been left with a pleasant glow. My cheeks feel rosy but I'm having to squint at the figures on the printout before me. Every so often the amounts double, then slalom across the green paper.

Tallying these figures forms a huge chunk of my life, from eight in the morning until sometimes nine in the evening. Monday to Thursday. Fridays tend to culminate in a more civilised 5 p.m. finish. Nine to five Saturday and Sunday.

On this floor of Edinburgh House in St Andrew Square, there are eight tables hosting teams of 14 clerks with one supervisor, each performing like workers in an ant colony. Another analogy would be comparing the tables to cogs in a machine: in one end the application forms requesting shares, out the other the letters confirming the number of shares allocated. Whether the customers are investing £50 for a minimum share, or thousands more, they will view these shares in terms of a way of increasing their original stake: capitalism as gambling, but with better odds than the Scottish National.

So we huddle over screeds of computer printouts, checking data against the information displayed on white ones. As each batch of green sheets is completed, errors marked by white stickers, it is secured by an elastic band and then passed to the bank staff for double-checking. When they uncover an anomaly lurking between those already flagged it is pounced upon with the vigour of crocodiles awaiting zebras by a waterhole. The printout is returned to its source to be thrust onto the table like an NFL touchdown, the mistake announced to the whole floor. Everyone knows these incidents are being recorded and will contribute to the decision about names to be culled during the next round of redundancies.

Poring over endless lists of names, addresses, and financial details, it is inevitable minds will wander. We banter, tell filthy jokes, goad each other, invent derogatory nicknames for our colleagues, and the bank officials. Sometimes the chattering ebbs and a sense of purposeful industry returns. At other times the gaggle rises to such a crescendo the team supervisors, the capos of this clerical world, must berate their staff and appeal for them to concentrate on the job at hand lest errors go unflagged.

If the supervisors are colluding in the banter, the bank staff will march across the floor and remind us all about the imminent P45s. This scenario is repeated across all the tables on this floor, and the others on the floors above and below.

Binge drinking becomes a major incentive, alcoholic oblivion the aura at the end of the tunnel of hours of drudgery. The thought of communal drunkenness is the imaginary carrot centermost in many of our minds, powering us through all these printouts until the moment the bank staff tell us when we can down pens and head downstairs to the Traveller's Tryst.

While there is some debate about the direction the subsequent pub crawl will take us, this Friday it's a foregone conclusion. The German beer tent is in town.

*

Queuing outside the canvas pavilion we joke about being the 'before' picture. We have a clear view of the 'after.' Every so often figures emerge from the arena of strident brass band music and raucous laughter, staggering when they hit fresh air. This is greeted with a roar as if they are lurching towards the finishing line to claim Olympic gold after a marathon.

One guy careers straight into bushes. Vomits. Two drunken mates materialise and plunge into the shrubbery to help him up. As this degenerates into a farcical scrum, we all egg them on. In the shadow of Edinburgh Castle, a looming fortress that endured 26 sieges in 11 centuries, here is a microcosm of Scotland's self-destructive love of alcohol, our perennial urge to lay siege to our livers and mental health.

Inside the tent, we are served huge schooners of potent lager. You pay a deposit that can either be reclaimed when you return the stein or forfeited if you take it away as a souvenir of the debauchery.

Much later I stumble through Princes Street Gardens, my sides and rump florid with bruises I'm too numb to feel after having fallen backwards from a long bench too many times to count. I focus on steering my uncertain footfall against the glaring daylight.

Every so often I halt, swigging the dregs from my Fursten-berg stein. Thrusting it above my head, an absurd trophy to damaged brain cells, my voice swirls.

Oh, Flower of Scotland ... when will we see...

My slurred lament echoes from the ramparts.

11

Too Many Screaming Orgasms

My pint feels more like a quart. As I raise it towards my parched lips its surface quivers, making me so self-conscious I place it back onto the Formica. Surrounding me are everyone else's empties. The rest of the company grew so impatient at my insistence I wasn't struggling with my drink they abandoned me. Clattering out Mister Mustard's to continue the session in Gatsby's. Now I glance around their glasses, replaying the conversation topics.

To my left, the dregs of Alex's McEwan's 80 shillings. He was describing last night's fancy dress pub crawl. One of the supervisors, Davie Pearson, nicknamed René due to his uncanny resemblance to the *'Allo 'Allo!* character, was dressed as Fidel Castro. At one point he was leading a conga down the Royal Mile.

Opposite, Splodge's lagers. Two glasses. He always demolishes his beers ahead of everyone, necessitating solo orders between rounds. We've all discovered the folly of trying to keep pace with him.

As Alex painted a picture of passers-by having to swerve out of the Cuban leader's way, Splodge gave him a shifty glance. That pair are always falling out. I've taken turns holding each of them back from going for the other. They're too alike – verbose, cocky, argumentative – never serious about anything beyond beer and their beloved boys in maroon. They're like two magnetic poles, always repelling.

Alex said René kept complaining about being so sweaty inside khaki fatigues and the stick-on beard he kept on having to adjust to tackle his beers. But for all he was spangled by the end of the night, he never lost that plastic cigar.

To my right, John's Tartan Special, the last third remaining. He seemed some distance from tempering his own hangover with that hair of the dog. At least he was attempting to, while my guts were churning.

I asked Alex who else was in the conga. When I lifted my drink, the head swilled overboard.

Splodge wagged a finger. Shaking like a leaf, Fleming. You're going to lose half that pint before it gets anywhere near your fucking geg. Bookable offence.

I managed a half-hearted smile to mask the more natural urge to wince. The vile liquid was so effervescent. I felt each rancid mouthful fizz all the way down, ballooning my belly.

Angela was a Rocky Horror Show nun, Splodge continued. John a *Wehrmacht* officer, complete with a fucking monocle. That was where the trouble started.

When I asked about this, Splodge rolled his sleeves up, taking centre-stage to recount the action.

Outside The Mitre, some prick took offence at John's getup, despite it being pointed out the costume was more *Hogan's Heroes* than *World at War*. He delved into the huddle of drinks for the second of those two empties, his fifth pint and it wasn't even 6 p.m. We clocked off at 5 p.m.

Splodge grinned as he outlined his own costume, Hitler, although this caused less offence because the parody was so obvious. His version of the Führer was the Freddie Starr interpretation. Shorts, wellies, and a tiny stick-on tache more reminiscent of Charlie Chaplin. He went on to delight in referring to Alex dressing like a tramp, the only person who hadn't bothered with fancy dress. Alex retorted, fuck off, he was a gentleman of the road.

Ignoring him, Splodge went on. Flapper girl, Samantha. Belly dancer, Mharaid. Elvis, Keith. Nell Gwyn, Nicola.

Spilling out everywhere by the end of the night, interrupted Alex. Splodge fired another look but colluded in smirking at the vision, before going on to mention Chris, a student from Boston near the end of the line. He was dressed as Harvey, the six-foot-tall white rabbit who was a figment of James Stewart's alcoholic imagination in the 1950 film. More than the occasional passer-by must have assumed they were similarly hallucinating towards closing time.

Taking up the rear was Donnie the quiet Hebridean, a Waterloo redcoat. He'd guzzled too many Screaming Orgasms in Styx and thrown up over his Napoleonic War medals.

Throughout this, I gripped my pint, studying the bubbles rushing to the surface. I pictured Donnie, lumbering around after overindulging on cocktails, his loquacious Isles accent becoming ever more unintelligible.

But the thought of the cocktail frenzy niggles my stomach. Reminds me of the previous Friday inside Styx. Alex was giving Nicola, an Australian temp, a high shoulder across the small dancefloor. She was facing him, skirts hoisted over his features, but not enough to prevent his impaired vision from noticing a stool. In a rare moment of responsibility, I lunged for Nicola's flailing limbs, only to create a cushion between Alex and the ground.

Later, as we were crossing Princes Street towards The Rutland, I spewed over the tarmac. Invoking groans and cheers. Minutes later I was immersed in the bar's boisterous hubbub, another lager before me.

Shuddering at the recollection, I remarked about so much debauchery during a sponsored pub crawl raising money for the Ethiopian famine appeal. Splodge acknowledged the irony, gulping more lager, patting his gut. At least they were doing *something* for the starving in Africa, not just pissing it all against the fucking wall.

I consider John's glass again. He launched into a fuller account of the scuffle. The prick began shoving him.

Game cunt, conceded Splodge, considering the dose of them in the company. The motley costumes maybe less intimidating.

John then mimed the action of his antagonist launching a hand at the collection tin he was holding. When he maintained a tight grip, the guy turned to Mharaid, demanding a private belly dance for him and his buddies down Bishops' Close, smacking her arse. Elvis, also a Hibs Boy in a more sinister alter-ego, nutted the lad. This lit the fuse to a wild but brief skirmish.

My queasy guts recoil at my next mouthful of the noxious phial of piss-coloured chemicals. I take deep breaths. A barman hovers, adding the glasses to a tray. I tell him my pint's dead, then head for the toilets. Entering a cubicle I slam the door, flip the lid down. Commence deep breathing.

Closing my eyes, I visualise the scene John described. Relieved I missed the senseless streetfight. Or was 'posted missing,' as Splodge kept goading me.

I imagine the conga weaving down the High Street. John making the most of his rented uniform, swaggering in grey jodhpurs and leather boots, a red rag to any of the drunken bulls crashing around the Old Town on a Friday night. Like most altercations incited by alcohol, the brawl would've been like a scene from The Keystone Cops, with misaimed punches instead of custard pies.

Nausea dissipates. I heave myself up and exit the cubicle. When I stood in this same position after my last slash, 15 minutes ago, Alex was next to me. He glowered into the mirror.

Fleming. Still got a full pint out there. Lagging behind, poof. Get your drinking head on, fuck sake. Long night ahead.

I shove my hands under the dryer. When I stroll by the empty table, I gaze out the window where I watched their riotous exit, Splodge, arms aloft, bellowing: *Para bailar la bamba!*

The thought of a pub crawl fills me with dread. This isn't just to do with my hangover from last night. I made some excuse. Just didn't feel like donning a ridiculous costume then waving a collection tin at randoms in High Street bars. Instead, I took refuge in my bedroom, Cocteau Twins, and Strongbow tins.

A lassie is quaffing a pint of cider. The notion puts me in mind of forcing down battery acid. I barge outside. Giddy. As if I've stepped off a roundabout. St Andrew Square is drenched in unforgiving sunlight.

To my left, I catch Alex hovering at the Gatsby's entrance, beckoning, before disappearing inside.

I turn to my right. A 44 is drawing into the bus stop. I break into an unsteady sprint.

12

Voices Of Reason

September 1987

Mum and Dad are doing dishes, discussing going to the Lyceum. Having popped round for lunch from work, Anne is fetching her jacket. My wee sister and I have always been close. I can discuss pretty much anything with her, expecting her to reciprocate. I've decided I'm going to level with her about the weird anxiety that's been creeping up on me. It might help to unburden my troubles.

Gearing myself up, I watch her poking her arms into the sleeves. I take a breath. Where will I start? The binge drinking and the late nights? The hangovers and struggling to drink coffee at work because my hands are such a blur? Or the job itself? The laborious slog of a 60-hour week of white-collar skivvying in a soulless office processing computer printouts, a vocation not so much dead-end as brain dead? The mood swings? My insomnia?

She hoists her handbag onto her shoulder. Smiling, she senses I want to chat, but my shiftiness is telegraphing this is for her ears only. I nod towards my bedroom, then follow her in, closing the door. Casting an eye over the walls, she comments you can still see the Blue-Tack marks. I visualise the poster display. Sham 69. The Vibrators. The Fall taking the lion's share of the available space. Posters, record sleeves, cuttings from *Sounds* and *NME*. *Everywhere.* Dad used to say it looked like the aftermath of a twister.

I flashback almost a decade to those brash, halcyon teenage days when picture sleeves were miniature works of art, far too expressive to be buried among stacks of similar seven inches. Everything from The Damned in their paper bag masks on the cover of 'Neat Neat Neat' to the iconic Jamie Reid design for The Sex Pistols' 'God Save the Queen' had formed the gaudy interior design to my room; mirroring many of my mates' bedrooms, and similar teenage lairs across the country.

But the stark white walls seem to reflect my present outlook. It's impossible to believe I once participated in a youth movement that celebrated anarchic music and zany fashion. Those picture sleeves are now stashed in piles gathering dust, the larger posters folded away in the loft. My hand-painted A2 facsimiles of The Fall's 'Bingo Master's Breakout' and PiL's 'Death Disco' picture sleeves will have long since yellowed.

Anne asks what's bothering me. Instead of answering, I just stare at the carpet. Although she's putting on a brave face, the edge to her voice tells me she's concerned. Where could I start? I haven't a clue. So instead of beginning to air my list of grievances I attempt to summarise, thinking of Splodge at work, the phrase he parrots on Mondays when he's decrying his weekend alcohol tally. *Finished*. So I tell her this. *I'm finished*.

What do you mean, *You're finished*?

When I repeat I'm finished, and that's all there is to it, she becomes more confused. Eyes welling. After taking a breath, it's her turn to unburden something that's been on her mind.

She starts by placing everything in context. I'm her big brother. She loves me but I'm scaring her. Do I realise how much I'm worrying Mum and Dad these days? They won't say as much to my face. They think I'm stressed out because of the job, and not taking enough time to chill between my weekend blowouts. Why do I think they've booked a holiday in Paris? I seem like a coiled spring, always on edge. They just want me to unwind. Revert to the boy they once recognised.

This is like a spell being broken, watching the wall of her innocence and unconditional love absorbing what probably came across as self-pity. I mumble something about not being myself, concluding I *do* need a holiday. The feeble backtracking has little effect. As she fixes me with her glistening eyes she looks unconvinced. I've created even more questions than gaining answers to whatever is bugging me.

But one thing I can grasp is that my confused mutterings are a symptom of something much deeper, a condition that in itself renders self-analysis impossible.

She envelops me in the type of embrace that always inspires embarrassed chuckles at Christmas or on birthdays but which is currently charged with emotion. As she heads out of my room, I tell her not to worry about me. But as I hear her shouting goodbyes to the folks, I appreciate how hollow my words must sound.

*

With the workload diminishing, the bank has paid off three-quarters of the temps. I've been showing up at work, getting through the day. The only outward sign of any deepening depression has been my increasing insularity.

Where I would once have been an enthusiastic participant, sometimes instigator, of post-work piss-ups, my social calendar is now empty. Colleagues merely read this as evidence of taking some timeout after a series of heavy weekends. In this binge drinking twentysomething subculture, reaching a level of alcohol abuse where regular drying out is necessary is regarded with kudos.

Returning from the office, I struggle to hold a conversation with my parents before tramping off to my room. I rifle through the paperbacks on my bookshelves, selecting HG Wells' *The Island of Doctor Moreau*. I used to devour fantasy fiction, and have read this novel more than once. Now I flip through the pages. Alighting on random paragraphs. Skimming the prose but not taking anything in. Treating classic literature in this way is the equivalent of strolling through the Royal Scottish Academy wearing sunglasses but I'm past caring.

The bedroom door opens. Mum hands me the portable phone. I demand to know who is calling me but she just hands it over, pre-empting any attempt to screen the call.

Flembo? I recognise my buddy, Grum. I used to say we manned the barricades together during the punk wars. That seems a lifetime ago. Chirpy as ever, he asks how I'm keeping. He says he was chatting with Alex, who told him the pair of us are working in an office in St Andrew Square. What's it like working with that mad Leither?

I could explain the work itself is mind-numbing. Working with a good mate means we can get a laugh, but the office environment's new to Alex. He spends as much time hovering around desks where he's pinpointed attractive girls. But it's easier to skulk behind a wall of apathy. I ramble I don't trust him or Alex anymore, mumbling about the pair of them ripping me off.

Dumbfounded silence. Then he adopts a different approach. Insisting we've been mates since school. He mentions how I came to every one of his gigs when he was fronting The Accidents. How I was once as mad about collecting vinyl as he was. Still is. He recognises I'm not myself at the moment. I'm going through something. He mentions someone in his family going through a tough period. A *breakdown*. Like the classic Buzzcocks song, he adds. Trying his best to lighten the mood. He wants to ask my mum a few questions.

I drop the phone. Pacing over to the window to stare into the back green, I can still hear him. But he now sounds so far away.

13

Head In The Clouds

October 1987

The night before the flight to Paris Charles De Gaulle my insomnia is off the scale. I'm glaring into the bedroom ceiling, trying to avoid fixating on my virgin flight in a metal cylinder 39,000 feet high.

Flying is a common enough phobia for healthy individuals. So what chance has someone with stress issues? The irrational fear of being atomized during a crash is eclipsed by the more tangible anxiety about letting my parents down when I admit I can't travel with them tomorrow, so the four-figure holiday cost is toast. This is the niggle that gnaws at me throughout the sleepless hours.

*

We are seated in the departure Lounge, Mum and Dad engrossed in *The Scotsman* crossword. I have a paperback opened across my lap, *The Fall of Kelvin Walker* by Alasdair Gray. But I can't concentrate on it. Instead, my attention is centred on four bottles of Holsten Pils clustered before me. My liquid anaesthetic.

Pinstriped men and women are seated at surrounding tables, noses buried in pink newspapers. Sipping coffee while discussing agendas and consultation fees. I'm aware of an occasional eyebrow being raised towards the young man throwing lager down his neck like a lone English football thug.

Given the rate at which I'm self-administering Dutch Courage, my eyes are watering and my guts are churning like a volcanic spring. When our boarding is announced I entertain the image of an inmate hearing the bolt grating on his Death Row cell door for the last time. I tank the dregs of the fourth bottle but fail to stifle a sound barrier-breaching belch. Mum fires a stare that could strip paint.

As we make our way to the desk, the family before us in the queue place my panic into its embarrassing context. Two adults hold hands with a boy and his sister, both under 12. The kids are watching planes taking off with a sense of wonder and excitement the polar opposite of my terror at watching 300 metric tons defying gravity. At least the alcohol is taking the edge off. Shuffling down the enclosed walkway to our waiting aircraft, I stumble into the wall. I snigger at this. Mum asks if I'm still feeling nervous. I scoff at the notion.

Onboard, the sight of other passengers chatting as if we're about to embark on a routine train journey relaxes me even more. I try not to dwell on the absurdity of buckling ourselves into seatbelts in case the plane should nose-dive to ground level from the troposphere.

The take-off is relaxed. Nothing like the experience I envisaged of a rollercoaster-like acceleration peeling back my cheeks. Moments later the landscape surrounding the airport has transformed with scale. Toy cars crawl along the M8. The Union Canal is a silver ribbon. Then clouds obscure the view while we climb towards cruising altitude.

I rubberneck at the flight attendant doing her safety dem-onstration, drawn to her choreographed routine but aghast at the way she mimes inflating the lifejacket and tugging out its little whistle. The prospect of surviving a ditching into the sea only reminds me of Quint's story in *Jaws* about shipwrecked US sailors inciting a feeding frenzy among sharks.

Thinking of the void metres below my feet makes my stomach flip. My parents, as unfazed as I am unhinged, and intent on a crossword, are seasoned flyers. Next year, they plan on travelling to Turkey to stay with Gokce, one of the English language students who once lodged with us. Dad will also fulfil a longstanding ambition to visit Gallipoli, between the Dardanelles Strait and the Aegean Sea. He's read umpteen histories on the prominent role that rugged peninsula played in World War 1, and has even brought one along for light in-flight reading.

The German lager has only dampened my paranoia, so I ask to borrow his book, burying my nose in this account of the 1915 military disaster.

The campaign began as a bold attempt by Churchill to open a second front to end the stalemate in France. The volume quotes the 40-year-old First Lord of the Admiralty: "The price to be paid in taking Gallipoli would no doubt be heavy, but there would be no more war with Turkey. A good army of 50,000 and sea power – that is the end of the Turkish menace."

Infantrymen jumping from ships to storm the beaches were strafed by machine guns on the clifftops, transforming the azure seas familiar with today's holidaymakers crimson.

The Allies lost 45,000 in the campaign's first months, and as they remained pinned down over 50% of the casualties were due to disease. *Dysentery*. A horrific inflammation of the intestines and colon caused by bacterial infection. Severe stomach cramps. Chronic diarrhoea, blood and mucus in the faeces. By tens of thousands, soldiers literally shat themselves to death. *Typhoid*. Another bacterial infection. Extremely swollen stomach. Headaches. Fever. Fatigue. More diarrhoea. As men lay untreated, they would lie with their eyes half-open, exhausted and delirious, in a semi-comatose position known as the typhoid state. *Trench Fever*. Spread by lice. Headaches. Dizziness. Muscle pain. Lesions. Although not as fatal as Dysentery or Typhoid, around one-third of the troops were infected. *Drowning*. Many of the volunteers who had viewed this patriotic adventure as an escape from inner-city slums had never learned to swim; entering the sea from ships, over-loaded with equipment, meant leaping into their own deaths. During the eight-month campaign, there were heavy storms in

October, flooding the trenches. *Heat*. Sunstroke would cause men's brains to swell, while artillery often set the dry scrub alight, engulfing the wounded and dying. *Cold*. As winter set in, snow, ice and blistering winds howled across the Sea of Marmara from Russia.

According to a Private Harold Boughton: "One of the biggest curses was the flies. There was millions and millions and millions of flies. The whole of the side of the trench used to be one black swarming mass. If you opened a tin of bully or went to eat a biscuit, next minute it would be swarming with flies. They were all around your mouth and on any cuts or sores that you'd got, which all turned septic through it."

Joseph Napier of the South Wales Borderers: "Lying between the trenches, you've never seen such an array of corpses and bodies and all stages of death and so on and colour and blowing up. And the flies were having a harvest of a time among these. Then of course they came into the trenches where food was being eaten and served. It was quite a job to get the food into your mouth before a fly got on to it."

Around 100,000 soldiers from all sides lost their lives. While all those telegrams and letters were being opened, from Perth in Perthshire to Perth in Western Australia, Ottowa to Ankara, Churchill was demoted, eventually resigning from the government.

Mum interrupts my history lesson, asking the hometown of the Scottish Cup holders. Paisley, I tell her. When one of the hostesses brings her rattling trolley along the aisle I request a gin and tonic.

I feed my Sony Walkman's earplugs in and switch on the cassette: *Treasure* by Cocteau Twins. The ethereal soundscapes synchronise with the fantastical visuals. Viewing the cloud canopy from above it appears as if we are drifting over a glacier stretching to the horizon. A gap reveals a patchwork quilt of fields and a symmetrical new town I assume to be Livingston. The jet wheels to the south, occasional tears in the cloud cover revealing the Southern Uplands, while Liz Fraser's fluid lilt exacerbates the dreamlike experience. My recent lack of sleep conspiring with the morning's breakneck alcohol consumption, I sink into slumber.

At one point I come to and realise I'm bursting for the toilet. I make my way to the cubicle. Inside, I try blotting out the notion of thousands of feet of nothing below my wobbling legs. That's when I notice it. I delve further, tugging the opening wider. A rash of red spots peppers my pubic hair. Payback for months of an alcohol-driven and lackadaisical attitude to my sleeping arrangements.

Swaying back to my seat I can think of nothing else. Should I make an appointment to see a French doctor? Do they even have the equivalent of the NHS? Can I delay this another few days until I'm back in Edinburgh?

As I dwell on the implications of ignoring my condition, my befuddled mind begins self-diagnosis. When you're part of a gang for whom unprotected sex is an occupational hazard, you goad anyone who gets caught out. Banter descends into euphemisms. Seaside nippers. A dose. The clap. But one-night stands in Edinburgh equate to a much more sinister condition. Edinburgh? AIDS capital of Europe.

My train of thought unravels for the remainder of the flight until the pilot announces we've started our descent. Mum indicates the fields and woods now hoving into view is *La France*.

Paranoia envelops me. A ferocious headache is mustering behind my teary eyes. The overhead signs are imploring everyone to clip their seatbelts. I peer outside, hoping to glimpse the remnants of the soothing carpet of cotton wool. The plane lurches below the clouds, ailerons flapping as it drops ever closer to impact.

14

Paris In The Autumn

Compared to Edinburgh Airport, Charles de Gaulle is gargantuan. Everything is a blur, the sensation overload compounding the pain inside my skull. Passengers bluster by, offering random snatches of the planet's 6,500 languages, luggage often employed as battering rams. Police scrutinise us all, sporting the shades they probably assume exude a potent combination of cool and toxic masculinity. Exemplified by toting submachine guns.

*

A grouchy driver watches me heaving our baggage into his boot, before setting off on what resembles a waltzer ride with a meter. Sucking from the Gauloise jammed between his lips, he peers over rimless glasses, muttering at every obstacle. Racing into dense traffic, whenever manoeuvrability seems impossible he manages to exploit the narrowest of gaps, weaving between buses and articulated lorries. Cutting down sidestreets and across lanes, his vehicle is a magnet for the horn blasts he dismisses with an emphatic shrug.

But window displays of boulangeries and patisseries get my mouth watering, and I spy the three white domes of the Sacré-Cœur, towering above Montmartre. When the driver deigns to obey a red light I marvel at the chic Parisians I observe congregating outside a café. Young and old, everyone is dressed to impress. Armani. Lacoste. Valentino. Aquascutum. Nicole Farhi. I suspect wearing a shellsuit is one of the few penalties that might still warrant the guillotine.

We arrive at the Hotel Genève in the 9th Arrondissement. After checking in we take the lift up to our respective rooms. Mum and Dad are on the top floor; I'm immediately below. We agree to unpack then meet in an hour to search for a café for an evening meal.

Alone in my room, I take stock. My head is still racing with all the sensations of travel. I glower out the window, hoping for a view over the city. Instead, I see the opposite flats, grey and weatherbeaten, as if nothing much has changed since someone stood in this spot anticipating air raid sirens in 1940.

After filling the wardrobe with my clothes, I stretch out on the bed. Open my paperback. I can't concentrate and have to re-read several paragraphs. In an attempt to focus I sit up and perch on the edge of the bed, flicking on the kettle. Mixing myself a cup of tarry French coffee all the milk cartons fail to discolour, I add five sugar sachets. I confront the pages again.

A crimson dot appears on the print, joined by several more in quick succession. My nose is bleeding all over the library book and the crisp white sheets. Staring at the ceiling I pinch the bridge of my nose until it stops. I remember the tip for countering blood spillage. Cold water. I douse everything in undrinkable Parisian tap water.

For the remainder of the hour, I gaze out of the window, observing pigeons squabbling on the rooftops, convinced the chambermaids will think me some kind of freak from Scotland. Carrying the Virus.

*

There's such an atmosphere to savour that in different circumstances I would've had a brilliant holiday. After rendezvousing last night we headed for a restaurant recommended by the reception staff, a local Algerian outlet. Ravenous after the long trip we tucked into couscous and mouth-watering lamb washed down with a full-bodied red. Today I'm just another tourist, one whose head is fuzzier than most of the others gawking and queuing.

Dad declines the trip to the first level of the Eiffel Tower but Mum and I head up, taking snaps of the magnificent iron structure, then studying the sprawling cityscape. Unlike Edinburgh viewed from a height, where you can see the Pentlands to the south or the Firth of Forth in the other direction, bleached white buildings stretch to the horizon from every compass point.

Later, we visit the Louvre, where Dad takes a shot of Mum and me sharing a joke by the Venus de Milo, taking our place in the similar poses that will nestle in photograph albums from Greenland to Tasmania. Awaiting the shutter click I grin but this seems to strain jaw muscles unfamiliar with this expression for so long.

Covering the visitor locations necessitates a great deal of underground train travel. Below ground, Dad pores over his map, pinpointing where we are in relation to the metropolis whizzing above us. He takes pride in his mastery of the colourful routes and his ability to decipher the various points where we can switch lines to optimise our journey. This skill was developed during years of London commuting after he was transferred from Ireland to the GPO Stores HQ in Studd Street, Islington. He first bumped into Mum in a civil service hostel in Wimbledon in the late 1940s, delivering the immortal opening line: *are you a wee Scots lassie?*

Although I'm putting on a front of displaying all the enthusiasm of a Parisian novice, I continue stoking my malaise. My depression wasn't abandoned at Edinburgh airport. It has accompanied me on this holiday like a dangerous stowaway, an ever-present darkness that no amount of delicious French cuisine or fabulous architecture will nullify.

Paranoia simmers. Seeps into my pores. Volatile as leaking gas. Heading towards a tube station I can't meet anyone else's gaze. My self-awareness has magnified. Mutated. I fire awkward glances into shop fronts crammed with tantalising food displays; some are less enticing, with whole hares strapped to hooks. All the time I sense I'm being scrutinised.

It's even worse on the Metro. Huddled into the claustrophobic carriages, the blur of the world outside the windows compelling everyone to focus on other passengers, I stare at my shoes. I'm convinced someone will realise I'm diseased.

An old woman sitting opposite is listening to Mum and Dad discussing The Louvre, no doubt speculating which part of the English-speaking world these visitors are from. She is about to point a wizened finger at me like a prosecution witness at Salem. *J'accuse.* I anticipate her merciless tone. Word will be passed around that an AIDS carrier is lurking in their midst.

The fact I'm plagued by these delusions only to emerge ignored and unscathed into Parisian daylight does nothing to pre-empt the next panic attack.

*

We book a cruise down the Seine. Gliding along the wide river we pass beneath a bridge. Someone has spray-painted under its arch's dark bricks: 'Bonjour Mamie'. Mum's name. This is no coincidence. The graffiti proves we are being stalked. Even as the boat drifts by the 35-feet replica Statue of Liberty, I know my every move is under scrutiny from the banks. Paris is watching.

15

First Confession In Paris

After trying snails for lunch, grateful the mouth-watering sauce diverted my attention from the thought of chewing creatures that leave slime trails, the folks go to buy postcards and a souvenir for Grannie.

I head off to meet Anne, who is staying at her boyfriend, Brian's flat. An English teacher who recently accepted a teaching job in Paris, he's also a jazz trombonist, and a member of Tam White & the Dexters. Tam is a longtime Edinburgh blues singer, the first-ever performer to sing live on *Top of the Pops* in 1975, and the gravelly voice behind Robbie Coltrane's Big Jazza McGlone in the recent BBC Scotland series *Tutti Frutti*.

A few weeks ago, Anne dropped the bombshell on our parents that she's planning to resign from being a secretary with the Scottish Investment Trust to relocate. She left for Paris before us to start getting familiar with her imminent new home.

She has provided directions to a bar she and Brian like. I've circled it on my fold-up map: the Kennedy Eiffel, 16 Avenue du Président Kennedy. She told me it's situated on a street corner on the River Seine's north bank, next to the Pont de Bir-Hakeim. I can't miss its red awning.

Taking a Tube to the 16th Arrondissement, I meet Anne already enjoying a glass of white wine at a table by the windows. A waiter wearing a waistcoat strides over, smiling while I gawk at the huge viaduct and the ceaseless parade of cars and trains traversing the river. I order a lager.

After the guy has presented a bottle of Kronenbourg 1664, along with a slender glass and a circular mat, he smiles and about turns, his shiny brogues squeaking. Once he's out of earshot, Anne informs me this bar featured in *Last Tango in Paris*. In the opening scenes, Marlon Brando's character, Paul, is pished in here, and he staggers off to throw up in the *toilette*. That barman is the head of the bar, *le chef barman*, and guested in the film, serving Marlon Brando. She laughs, adding she doubts many of my mates in Edinburgh can say they've been served beer by someone who also served Marlon Brando.

Colluding with the notion, I grin, decanting the chilled lager. But my mirth is short-lived. I gaze into the bubbles rising inside my glass. It must appear as if I've got something on my mind again because Anne pauses, taking a sip from her wine. I look up. I want to divulge *everything*.

I have a bombshell of my own to drop on the family, a nuclear missile compared to Anne's firework about moving to Paris, and my opening salvo is going to be directed at her.

I want to explain I know I'm ill. I've felt ill for weeks now. I'm paying for a lifestyle that, while hardly Led Zeppelin-level hedonism, is still far beyond anything our parents ever went through. Copious alcohol. Unprotected sex with women as loose as me. That I'm sure I've contracted the HIV that will condemn me to a lingering death.

People with this condition are sacked without any hope of an appeal, ostracised within their communities. In North York-shire, rather than a respectful burial, a victim was entombed in concrete. In Florida, haemophiliac kids who had tested positive for AIDS antibodies, but not the disease, were banned from their school, their homes firebombed. I read about a poll in Los Angeles where the majority of respondents thoughts AIDS sufferers should carry identity cards and be quarantined. Because there is no cure, paranoia is rampant; rather, paranoia's retarded twin, ignorance, like 1987's answer to the McCarthy witch hunts. This will all break my family's heart.

I've rehearsed this spiel in my head, over and over, and poor Anne is will be burdened with it before anyone. My confession will begin flowing after I've blurted out the introduction. That should be easy enough to articulate. I just need to be honest, as if this table in a waterfront tavern is a confessional booth. My lager's effervescence might focus my pinballing thoughts. The tiny trails almost look purposeful, as if being driven by some intelligence. Lager relies on yeast, a single-celled organ-ism, a fungus. My resolve evaporates like the bubbles reaching the surface.

Anne begins chatting about how much she's looking forward to becoming a Parisian, taking French classes. I gaze into her cheery face. How could I burst that bubble? I decide to postpone my heart-to-heart, leave the metaphoric bomb ticking away. But when I catch up with Mum and Dad back at the hotel, that's when I'll detonate it.

*

Dad has been suffering from intermittent back pains for several years. Aggravated by all the walking and stair climbing of the past few days, this has recurred with a vengeance. When I pop up to their room he's prostrate on the bed, in agony, numbing himself with large Cointreaus. Outside, Montmatre is being battered with stair-rod rainfall.

We watch the TV showing *Les Vacances de M. Hullot*. There are no sub-titles but slapstick crosses national boundaries. Despite the anti-climactic sense of having visited the French capital only to spend our last night watching a film, the three of us enjoy it, although my giggling is so much more half-hearted than my parents, longstanding fans driven to uproarious laughter by many scenes.

As the credits roll, Mum pops down to the hotel foyer to buy water. I opt to keep the patient company, although I'm nobody's ideal conversational partner at the moment. Considering the prospect of paranoid mumbling interspersed with protracted silences, Dad demolishes his latest Cointreau, places the glass next to the bed. Within minutes, he's snoring.

I'm thinking about my confession. The one I was going to broach with Anne first because I thought it would be easier with her. But couldn't. I'll reveal all to Mum when she returns. After I've poured myself a Cointreau or two. Actually, do I *really* want to ruin the last night of the holiday? Maybe I'll wait until we get back to Scotland.

In the meantime, I need to butter them up. I dig into my jeans and withdraw a wad of currency, the remains of my holiday float. I count out 520 Francs, then pace over to one of Dad's jackets hanging in the wardrobe, bundling the notes inside a side pocket.

Afterwards, I stare at the screen, tap the remote, flicking through the channels until I discover football. There's a clip from the recent derby, Racing Club beating Paris St-Germain 2-1, the impartial commentator reacting to a late consolation goal by PSG as if he's just scooped a million Francs in a casino. Dad's snoring intensifies.

16

Sinking

Passengers are bowed over magazines or peering out at the English Channel far below, the world's busiest shipping lane reduced to a greenish-grey expanse with dots. The dread and guilt gnawing at me for so long were abated by becoming immersed in the colours, sounds, and scents of Paris. Now, returning home, my condition's temporary time-out is over, replaced with a renewed and invigorated sense of despair. The nonchalant voices surrounding me cast this into stark relief.

Fumbling into the pouch behind the seat in front, I dig out a glossy brochure. Flicking through, I discover safety instructions. Images of an aircraft that has ditched in the sea. Cartoon smoke pluming from its fuselage. In a close-up, a female blows into a whistle. Over the decades, how many times has a shrill squeak amongst welling waves saved a life?

Surely optimism doomed to failure. Reminds me of a documentary about early attempts at flight I once watched.

Franz Reichelt, a tailor, designed a parachute costume. Despite warnings and a broken leg after a trial jump from a window, he insisted his invention would immortalise his name. Juddery footage captured his moment of glory. Waiting to capture a gust, he stepped to the edge of the Eiffel Tower's first platform from a rickety chair. Instead of a graceful descent into the history books, pages ahead of Bleriot and the Wright brothers, he was pulped into Paris 187 feet below. Imagining *The Sun* headline almost brings a smile. Dickarus.

The doomed woman in the graphic also reminds me of a story Dad told me. An Irish friend, Danny, accommodated in the same civil service hostel in Wimbledon, was returning home in January 1953 on the car ferry *Princess Victoria*. Despite gale warnings, the vessel sailed for Larne, only to sink after the sea breached the stern doors. Danny was one of the 133 who drowned. Of the 44 survivors, none were women or children. So soon after the war, it appeared the 'men second' stiff upper lip had been in short supply during the terrible scramble for the lifeboats.

Dad pointed him out in a group photo, beaming to the camera with curly hair and glasses. I visualise Danny in cartoon form, having fitted into his snug lifejacket, in the icy North Channel, bobbing among the massive waves, surrounded by scores of passengers and crew in lifejackets, each coming to terms with their destinies. Perhaps he was imagining Dad singing 'Danny Boy' to him. Dad admitted he would regale him with the song's opening line towards closing time.

As I poke the brochure back, another thought slithers into my mind. I was 10, on holiday, playing in Coldingham Bay. The sea was choppy so people were clambering aboard lilos to surf towards the shore. A large wave caught me off guard and separated me from my lilo.

Arms thrashing, I tried touching the sand with my feet. I'd also been dragged out of my depth. As a non-swimmer this notion was terrifying. Another wave battered me and I gulped an acrid mouthful of salty water. Coughing and spluttering, I panicked. Then I stopped panicking. For a moment, a fleeting moment, I contemplated: this was the end. With this realisation, the anxiety dissolved into weird calmness.

But I spied my cousin Ross anticipating the next sizeable wave. I shouted on him. Oblivious to my predicament, he glanced in my direction, more in annoyance. Then I shrieked for help. Ross swam towards me. Grasping an arm, he hauled me into the shallows. Those feelings, panic and unnatural calm, faded into overwhelming relief.

*

In Heathrow Airport, I'm heading to the toilets. I leave Mum and Dad in the waiting area, drinking coffee, and keeping one eye on the departures for Edinburgh. During my labyrinthine quest to follow the signs to the Gents, I gaze over the airport's vast concourse. My latest absurd notion is this. I could start a new life here. Find the closest Tube station. Join the thousands who get swallowed by the metropolis annually. I could get casual work. Buy new clothes. Grow my hair. Change my name.

I also appreciate many of my fellow Scots, enticed by London's bright lights like moths to a flame, have been burned. Surrendering to alcohol and/or drugs. Being exploited or abused. Ending up on the streets. The idea dissipates. I imagine altering one's identity takes considerable planning and, even more crucially, some sense of optimism for a rebooted future. Each of these factors rules me out.

*

On the journey's final stage, the taxi ride from Edinburgh airport. I gaze out at familiar streets. But they have never looked so terrifying. My folks justifiably assumed Paris would help chill me out. Ease my stress. It's had the opposite effect.

After unpacking, I stare out the front room window. The prospect of venturing out there fills me with dread. I think of Janice, the trainee accountant, am consumed with shame for having sneered at her predicament. My hollow words have come back to haunt me. Assuming mental issues can be countered by the patient giving themselves a metaphoric shake, what alpha males might grunt about 'growing a pair,' is pathetic.

Someone else who went way beyond the point of being shaken back to normality was Daniella, another story treated with scepticism when I heard it from Mum at the dinner table. The older sister of one of the kids my Auntie Mary teaches at Towerbank Primary in Portobello, Danni dropped acid at a party. Instead of coming back down after a few hours, she lingered in a paranoid limbo for days, ending up in a psych ward.

You aren't aware of the extent of these individual tragedies because mental ill-health seeps below society's radar, burdened by stigmatisation, the stark truth dissipated by gibes about being carted away in 'the yellow van.' But whether they're prompted by one bad trip, or in my case, a creeping affliction, the final crash perhaps years in the making, the result can be catastrophic for the subject and those close to them.

Now I'm recalling a line manager from the Scottish Widows. Iain Dalgleish. When we convened to The Southern for lunchtimes pints, he would unleash impressions of just about anyone from the office you cared to tee up for him. He sometimes spent the entire hour or so conversing according to a particular theme, everything from pop stars to football managers. He once had me helpless with laughter after haranguing a drunken nuisance in the voice of Bill Shankly.

That was another of his passions, Liverpool FC. Iain had a red and white striped scarf draped from his desk. Lovingly described himself as a Silverknowes Red, his proudest experience was playing golf with Kenny Dalglish and Graeme Souness at a charity event. He wore a white Club Brugge shirt to work social events, a souvenir of attending the 1978 European Cup final at Wembley.

Iain gave every impression of being 100% healthy. Right up until the Friday afternoon when he clocked-out to embark on his usual weekend of football and DIY. None of us ever saw Iain again. He parked in his garage but left the engine running. He left behind a mystery more perplexing to his wife and teenage kids than where the universe ends.

17

Witch Trials

Although we got back from holiday a week ago, I haven't returned to work. Mum is phoning the office with an update. I listen at the door. She mentions forwarding my latest sick note, followed by an update after my next GP appointment.

I retreat to the dining room. Dad's in the bathroom. Shaving. *Radio 2* blaring. I prise open the drinks cabinet. Tug out a bottle of QC. Slug a mouthful. This syrupy drink once had a powerful medicinal effect, curing hangovers within a few sips. Thanks to my medication the mouthfuls just render me nauseous.

Throughout my later teens and early 20s, sleep was the other counter to the side effects of weekend binges. The flexible Napier timetables meant early lectures could be skipped. This was perfect for the lifestyle I was leading, the boozy band practices and gigs embodying the spirit of the times. My course, Publishing, was a hotbed for local indie music, the year below me spawning The Shop Assistants, Rote Kapelle, and Jesse Garon and the Desperadoes.

But a year has passed since I was a student who could drink to all hours any night of the week, then use 'home study' as a lie for lie-ins. My vague aim of embarking on a career connected with my qualification evaporated long ago.

A few days before we left for Paris, I was addressing share acceptance certificates. Discovered my pen vibrating in my fingers, then my whole hand trembling. Attempting to concentrate on my task, gripping the implement tighter, only made this worse, the text now indecipherable. Sweat prickled my brow. My pulse drilled. The sight of everyone surrounding me methodically printing out the required information accentuated my panic attack

I put the pen down and headed to the toilets. Locked myself in a cubicle, deep-breathing. But I couldn't shake off the feeling I'd just clambered from a waltzer. I knew I wouldn't be able to carry on.

Back at my desk, I willed my hand to cease its remorseless quivering before a coffee break was announced at 11 a.m. I joined Splodge, John, and Alex in the Traveller's Tryst. Four rounds, four nips each. When I returned I completed my forms with the fastidious attention of a monk scribing the Domesday Book.

Splodge got it right. The Traveller's Tryst was the cure to everything. Boredom. Hangovers. So many guys at work think that way. I used to.

*

I'm rummaging through *Sounds* cuttings, then scrunching them into the bin. I skim a review of *Live At The Witch Trials* headed, "Music for the man who has everything." Ten years old, it's yellowing. I feel as if I have nothing.

I flinch when the phone rings. I make out Mum chatting, before calling for me. The door opens. Mum passes the phone. Alex, she says. But I mumble I'm not up for talking. Cupping a hand over the mouthpiece, she insists he just wants to chat.

I take the portable phone from her. Alex asks how I'm getting on, where I've been hiding, enthusiasm spilling 10 to the dozen in a Leith accent recognisable from so many glorious nights out, drunken singalongs, merciless banter, brilliant laughs, waxing lyrical about our shared musical passions, from The Skids to Roxy Music. Sharon at work's having her 18th at Sinatra's. I'm expected to be there. Her pal Tanya is hoping for an introduction.

I hang up.

*

I become engrossed in the screen. Among the adverts is a recurring health warning. A man struggles out of bed. Thin legs shamble along a corridor. Bare soles trembling as they contact linoleum. He finds a sink and a mirror. Staring at someone he no longer recognises.

Later, a far more foreboding variation to this theme. John Hurt provides a voice-over, gravelly tones intoning a message while a sculptor carves the word AIDS from a monolithic tombstone.

There is now a danger that has become a threat to us all. It is a deadly disease and there is no known cure. The virus can be passed during sexual intercourse with an infected person. Anyone can get it, a man or a woman. So far it's been confined to small groups, but it's spreading. So protect yourself and read this leaflet when it arrives. If you ignore AIDS it could be the death of you. So don't die of ignorance.

In my turbulent mind, a nonsensical connection. This advert is about me. The disease is rife in Edinburgh, not among the community stigmatized by the horrid 'gay plague' headlines in *The Sun* and *Daily Mail*. It is infesting the peripheral schemes where heroin addicts have been driven to share needles. My warped imagination is conjuring a fantastical chain of infection. A West Granton shooting gallery to a house party to a Lothian Road club. Ending right here, with me.

18

Vampires And Zulus

The doctor scribbling 'stress' on my medical certificates seems so inadequate. Having become agoraphobic, my anarchic imagination has transformed the outside world into a twilight zone where neighbours are conspiring to have us evicted, Mum has been threatened at the shops, and former friends are gophers for drug barons.

There are isolated moments when these delusions stall. Channel 4 shows black and white films in the afternoon. I find myself absorbed. Not by the plots which drift over my head but by the gentle pacing and affable dialogue, interspersed with melodrama. In the war films, the actors use three accents: public school English for the officers, Cockney for the other ranks, *Commando* comic German for the villains.

At tea-time, I still relish favourite meals. But these occasional rises in my bipolar graph are cast into stark relief by the frequency of troughs. And my burgeoning illness has become defined by one overwhelming symptom. Insomnia. Abject, red-eyed, morale-sapping insomnia. As the autumn sun begins sinking beyond Craiglockhart Hill, I know it is waiting for me, lurking in the deepening shadows. Moments of fitful slumber snatched on the settee during daylight only accentuate its terrible power. And no pills ever come close to vanquishing my nightly nemesis.

Tonight is no different. My latest mental torture session commences when I finally tear myself away from the TV's hypnotic spell. After gawking at *Hill Street Blues* I mumble goodnight. Mum and Dad repeat their well-worn mantra. They hope I'll get a decent night's sleep this time. Things will seem brighter in the morning.

I shamble through to my bedroom. Begin rummaging through papers. Receipts. Notebooks. Last year's college coursework. Rejection letters for short stories submitted to publishers. I sift through the latter.

I've never noticed how many there were until now. *New Edinburgh Review. The Scotsman. New Literary Review. The Stand. Granta.* Although I hoarded these as an incentive, many of the replies containing constructive criticism, I now see them for what they are: an accumulation of failure.

There are also crumpled letters addressed to my parents I retrieved from the bucket earlier. I'm looking for clues. Reasons I'm so hated. Once I've finished rifling through it all, I toss sheets around, creating a vast pile on the floor. I freeze. Rooted to the spot, I stare into the walls. Stoking my gloom. Impaled by guilt over everything I imagine responsibility for.

Mum pops her head round the door. Wondering if I've nodded off with the light on. I lie. I'm tidying. Don't want this weird inertia to faze her.

Weeks of sleeplessness have eroded my days and nights, so I don't even bother undressing. Lying on my bed in a T-shirt and jeans, I switch off my bedside lamp. A security light blazes from the Cowan Road tenements over the back greens. Cowering in the darkness, I stare at the way it shines through the gaps in the curtains. Casts a sliver of light against the wall. My warped perception gives this vision an added twist.

I'm now inside a Hammer film. A lynch mob mustering. Targeting the evil presence. My self-loathing has dragged me to such depths I'm now equating my existence with a vampire. But this illusion has an even more ludicrous distortion.

Among all the TV I'm reduced to ogling at as my sole leisure activity, I caught a news item about English football hooligans. There was a montage of the all-too-familiar clips. Pitch invasions. Rioting behind terracing partitions. Outside pubs. On station platforms. Footage depicted dawn arrests. Sheepish men were escorted from suburban houses, past kids' chutes, towards waiting police wagons. Some wore Burberry scarves tugged up to their furtive eyes like the outlaws they saw in their little minds' eyes when posing in front of mirrors, or before mates' disposable cameras on inter-city trains. Others attempted bravado, masticating gum while leering at the film crews. The commentary described ensnaring members of the self-styled Zulu gangs whose pointless campaign of hitting other grown men was done in the name of Birmingham City.

This lodged in some corner of my imagination. A posse of these Zulus have made their way from the Midlands. Now they're encamped in a flat overlooking my bedroom. They are responsible for directing this light towards my window every night. Their vigilante beacon. What this activity might instigate is irrelevant. I just accept being at the centre of it, a notion no more fanciful than any of the other gibberish clogging my mind.

As a break from my interminable tossing and turning, I heave myself from the duvet. Skulk over to the curtains. Anticipating lithe silhouettes darting to and fro, my trembling fingertips prise the curtains apart. I see their sinister searchlight.

I have to blink but it is trained on the bedroom that has become my cell, its beam as remorseless as the fantasies swirling inside my head.

19

Crazy Crazy Crazy
Crazy Guy

Flicking through the photo album, I dwell on the Easter photos. Mum and Dad have organised these family portraits every Easter Sunday since April 1963. The shots are always taken from the same vantage point, Anne and I seated on the piano stool.

In the inaugural one, I'm perched on Mum's lap. I'm on my own in the next, three months short of my second birthday. By the following year, my sister has arrived. And so the 12-month interludes continue, time distilled into a series of fashion lurches. Matching jerseys hand-knitted by Dad. Garish designs in tone with the 1970s wallpaper in the background. Gaps in teeth that mar cheeky smiles. Different hairstyles, especially Anne's, plunging to her waist, retreating to shoulder length.

As late 1970s/early 1980s teenagers, the clothes fluctuate. Anne's perms and Ra-Ra skirts. My punk spikes and Dennis the Menace mohairs. Easter 1985, two years ago, my mullet is resplendent.

The piano stool montage is such a simple idea. As a visual diary, it is priceless. If fire ever engulfed the house, this would be the first item I'd snatch. As I pore over it, I am engulfed with grief. This succession of beaming faces, especially in the early pages, represents innocence, a time when I had no concept of what lay ahead.

Visualising these snapshots as windows, I imagine what would assail my senses if I could travel beyond the limits of the frames. In my mind, I do just that.

I'm at the breakfast table in my Craiglockhart tie, listening to Dad's radio: Stravinsky's 'Rite of Spring,' the theme to *The Lost World*. He left much earlier for his new job in the GPO supplies depot in Newhouse, Lanarkshire. He commutes every day.

At the time I was obsessed with dinosaurs, asked for annuals at Christmas, collected pictures for a scrapbook from Crosse & Blackwell baked beans tins. My imagination conjures the giant predatory reptiles far more effectively than the film version, where the triceratops was some zoo lizard with prosthetic horns.

Hearing Dad returning from his long drive, I crawl beneath the sideboard to hide and he pretends he had no notion I might be in the same hiding place. Day after day.

Now I'm in my Tynecastle tie. Munching on toast lavishly spread with Mum's homemade crab apple jam, courtesy of her close friends, Margaret and Derek's back garden in Auchter-muchty. My nose buried in *Lord of the Rings*.

I enter my bedroom. Study posters of medieval battles from *World of Wonder* magazine. Trigan Empire strip cartoons from *Look and Learn*. The *Evening News* souvenir poster of Hibernian's 1972 League Cup triumph. In the background, our pet gerbils, Pixie and Dixie are gnawing the bars of their cage.

Now I'm in the front room, watching TV, the flickering box that lures me into more wondrous worlds. *Banana Splits. The Flashing Blade. Journey to the Centre of the Earth. The Golden Voyage of Sinbad.* Jon Pertwee fighting Daleks. Demons. Giant maggots. Sea devils. And a monstrous doll that came alive when heated, condemning Anne and me to nightmares.

I wander down the stairs. Out into the street where me and my pal opposite, Michael Malone, who goes to St Cuthbert's, the local RC school, play football for hours, always scoring against England at Wembley. The ball thumps against a window and an irate neighbour appears, Mrs Hunter, her pinched features reminding us of the witch from *Wizard of Oz*.

Chuck some water over the fucking faggot! Michael cries before we scamper into his house. His dad's got a single by Robin Hall and Jimmy MacGregor called 'Football Crazy.' Michael's not allowed to touch the record player, but when his dad's out at his work as a butcher, we play it and jig around the living room, kicking cushions around. His dad once told him Hall's ancestor is the Scottish outlaw, Rob Roy. That's how we like to play football. Like outlaws would.

When the Malones got their loft floored, Michael moved his bedroom up there. It's like our gang hut. We hang out with the third member of our inseparable trio, Alan Gray from number 10, surrounded by posters of Joe McBride, Pat Stanton, Eric Stevenson, and Peter Marinello. And cuttings from *Victor* and *Commando* comics.

We also play football all the time in the Craiglockhart playground. When anyone scores, we emulate Motherwell's Willie Pettigrew in the TV clip, kissing his boot from a standing position. Nobody ever manages it. When I stumbled into the railings, my mate Ian told me I was Fleming the drunk flamingo.

Further back, I'm at Mrs Calendar's sweetie shop on the way back from lunch, buying a sherbet fountain and Bazooka Joes with a threepenny bit. My pals, Ian, Barry, Crowie, Sparky and I are taking turns to do that Harry Worth trick, stretching our arms and legs against the shops' plate-glass windows.

We're in the school playground, swapping bubble-gum football cards. Joe McBride. Billy McNeill. Peter Cormack. Donald Ford. Colin Stein. Bushy sideburns and ragged fringes make them look as if they're about to pull stockings over their features before robbing a bank rather than gracing a football pitch.

Later, I feel I'm not a kid anymore when I'm allowed up for the Bells at Hogmanay. Drink two pints of shandy without being sick.

One of my keenest recollections doesn't feature in any of these snaps. But my first crush is seared into my memory. Melanie Green, from Mrs Nichol's class. A family joke revolved around the time I came home from Craiglockhart and announced Melanie and I were going to be married. We'd made all the arrangements. Reinforcing this sentiment, I made Valentine cards for Mum, Dad and Anne, with scribbled redcoat soldiers on each, and the legend, "I love you, and Melanie Green." I must've been about seven.

I sit with the pages opened in 1969, when the rest of the world was focusing on Vietnam and that Giant Leap for Mankind. Soon the photographs are shimmering through my tears.

Mum comes into the room with a tray of coffee and biscuits. She ponders my glum expression. Tells me she thought the album might cheer me up. I can't begin to explain why it has had the reverse effect.

*

The new Kiss single is blasting from the radio. *These are crazy, crazy, crazy, crazy nights.* This is the third time I've heard it today. The guys at work keep requesting it. I let it slip I was a Kiss fan in my mid-teens. They're noising me up. They know I'm ill, reclusive. They're *goading* me.

Tina, the American student from the office, is a New Yorker. Tina is a notch on Gene Simmons' bedpost. The guy's alter-egos are Dr Love. The Demon. The God of Thunder. Playing the part involves lurid make-up. A protruding tongue. Armour. Stack-heeled boots. Coughing up stage blood. Fire-breathing. A demonic deity is bound to be a sexual predator, and the Republican-voting rocker born Chaim Witz brags of conquests running into the thousands, and of possessing polaroid mementoes of each.

Tina is more than another one of his glossy shagging souvenirs. She has told him all about me. As well as being a walking culture for every STD under the sun, he has outspoken rightwing sympathies. That's why he's rejigged the lyrics. To out me as a certifiable pinko ex-punk. He'll make me rue the day I ever tore down my *Kiss Alive II* posters and replaced them with The Ramones. Now they are singing, *He's a crazy, crazy, crazy, crazy guy*. Kiss are broadcasting this to the world. Mark Fleming is mad.

20

The Stationary Sixties

Gawking into the mirror is like Dorian Gray coming across his portrait. The hair I once sculpted with hairsprays, gels, and mousse resembles something growing by a railway line. The eyes are glazed. The bags beneath are a testament to my non-sleep pattern. I wonder how I got to this. I was another twenty-something office drone living for the weekend. Binge-drinking wasn't a problem. It was a synonym for socialising.

I was also a greedy participant in what is aptly described as 'casual' sex: the exchange of names often an afterthought to that of bodily fluids. I endured the hangovers and the rationed sleep because the next binge was hours away. Less with Dad's drinks cabinet.

I can't face any more partying. I can't face *anything*. This is my existence. Self-imposed exile. I've given up on my job, my social circle. Leisure time translates as mind-numbing daytime TV, followed by nightly insomnia. Mum keeps explaining the doctor's lines. About my being signed-off work with a stress-related illness. But I can't grasp what this means anymore. I haven't just retreated in a physical sense. I've reverted to feeling like a child. My parents try to deal with my illogical behaviour as best they can. But in an era where information about mental breakdowns amounts to fading pamphlets handed over by the GP they have few reference points. Their recourse is to treat my delusional nonsense as if I've regressed to childhood.

Last night I caught *Top of the Pops*. Once staple viewing that signposted my growing up, from glam to rock, punk to electronica and house. Presented by Mike Smith and Gary Davies in jackets with their sleeves rolled up like I used to do, it was a garish meld of cheesy chart hits against a backdrop of constant, epilepsy-inducing, flashing lights.

One video was for 'Walk the Dinosaur' by Was Not Was, the dancers wearing faux animal skin bikinis aping Raquel Welch in *One Million Years B.C.* One girl was the double of a nurse I was seeing a few months back. Judy. At one point I was convinced it *was* Judy. Gyrating. Taunting. Every hip thrust emphasizing my libido is flat as a cardiograph plugged into a corpse.

*

I have slipped through a time warp. As I am cajoled into Dad's car, lower lip jutting like a petulant brat, I am convinced I am re-living my childhood. When Mr Brown shuts his gate, waves at Dad then sets off whistling, he is also re-enacting a moment from years ago. I notice Miss Cameron at number 12, peering out her window. Catching Dad's eye, she grins. Another neighbour is bowed over his van's open bonnet. My appearance has been everyone's cue to perform.

We pass the shops Mum took me around as a kid. I visualise the store where we bought tins of Heinz baby foods for my sister. Adams the grocer, who I confused with Captain Kirk, working his bacon slicing machine. Mac's the Greengrocer on the corner and towards Harrison Park, Brownsmith's, supplier of recruits for my Airfix armies. Shoppers. A postie. A window cleaner. All role-playing.

The surgery's interior hasn't altered much since the late 1960s. The posters on the waiting room wall mention polio jabs, breast cancer, STDs: timeless ailments. Dr Patterson pokes his head around the door. Although I receive a fleeting impression of trademark glasses and balding hair, I see him as I did decades before, the man Mum called out to the house in days of mumps, measles, and chickenpox.

Today I'm not seeing Dr Patterson. I'm seeing Dr McCabe. When my name is called, Mum escorts me into the surgery. Explains how I think I've picked up a serious sexually-transmitted disease. She baulks at mentioning AIDS. Perhaps Dr McCabe ponders about a grown man's self-diagnosis being introduced by his mother. But something about the way he raises his attention from the folder containing my medical notes makes the ridiculous scenario all too plausible. When she adds I've been prescribed anti-depressants by my regular GP, Dr Patterson, he nods.

He says, I see that, Mrs Fleming. Amitriptyline. That's fine, thanks for filling me in. If you'd like to take a seat in the waiting room again, I'll check Mark out. He's in good hands.

Aghast at Mum being forced to take control, I'm also relieved. Anything approaching a lucid explanation is way beyond me. I mumble replies to his earnest queries about the nature of the lice rash my paranoia has blown out of all proportion. He asks me to drop my trousers. As he fingers through the wiry hair with his rubber gloves, peering through a telescopic device, ever more absurd notions flit through my mind.

His calm manner. His wire-rimmed glasses. A front. His affable demeanour is masking an air of menace. Then it occurs to me who he reminds me of. Callum Kelso, a guy who used to bully me.

On the way back from primary school, Kelso would pin me to the wall outside his house. *Wait here, Fleming. I'm going to drop off my school stuff, come back out, punch your fucking lights out.*

For emphasis, his finger would slice across his throat. I would stand there. Sheepish. He would compel me to stay where I was, like a hypnotist weaving his spell, touching his neck. As soon as he disappeared, I would scamper away. This private vignette played out for several days until he must've got bored with returning to discover his prospective punchbag gone.

I also know this humiliating strip search is being filmed by a hidden camera. When he dismisses me with a prescription for antibiotics and cream, his imagined laughter rings in my ears. I return to the car. We stop off at the local chemist for the prescription. Applying the cream in the bathroom I know it won't cure the AIDS my mind is insisting is corrupting my blood. As for what today's date, month, or year might be, I haven't the faintest idea.

21

The Chingford Skinhead

The TV is beaming the Tory party conference from Blackpool. Norman Tebbit is addressing the audience. His haggard and humourless features remind me of a younger Peter Cushing. Except there's no endearing twinkle in these eyes. In the flesh, he's even more intimidating than his thuggish puppet on *Spitting Image*.

He stares into the camera. I flinch. Although he's referring to an autocue, I know the score. When he states the main thing restraining the economy is the prevalence of shirkers, it's not for the benefit of his middle-aged, Middle English congregation. It's for me. He's talking *to* me. *Blaming* me. I've become his sole focus. Any moment he's going to mention my name.

Glancing outside the window I notice two bricks on the walls of the house opposite. Sooty in colour. During Tebbit's tirade, they've been activated. They're stereo speakers. As the

Tory Chairman rails against me, his sunken eyes following me, these twin amplifiers are channelling his diatribe across the back greens, over the surrounding streets.

I march into the kitchen where Mum is rinsing dishes. She asks if I'm okay. When I tell her I'm anything but okay, she asks why. I tell her the score. I'm going to hand myself in. When her eyebrows arch, I try to explain I'm going to hand myself in to the police. Torphicen Street station is closest. I'm going to do this because of what Norman Tebbit has just told me. I'm a malingerer. I heard it through the PA system in Almondbank Terrace. And when I was in the bathroom earlier, I heard someone on the roof. Inserting bugging devices.

That she humours rather than laughs at me indicates how wary she is of the nonsense I'm liable to spout these days. In truth, she would have been adopting this lucid approach to mask her despair.

Mum shuts her eyes. Mustering a smile, she breaks the news they've made another appointment with the doctor. This deepens my paranoia. I blurt out my feelings about him. I've told her before. Dr McCabe *isn't* Dr McCabe. I saw the Burberry scarf draped from his surgery door. Terracing chic.

She ignores this. More lighter-hearted, she suggests I channel my fertile imagination into writing again. She reminds me of the short stories published in our local newspaper, the *Gorgie Dalry Gazette*. She remembers the story about someone getting thrown out of a pub in St Andrew Square. Written in the first person, she adds, grinning. Or science fiction? Didn't

I co-write a novel with my school friend, Brian? Did we ever finish it? Why not get in touch with Brian and pick up where we left off?

I know what she means by a *fertile imagination*. She might as well have tapped the side of her head.

*

I'm refusing to go. I hear Dad's clumsy approach from their bedroom. His back pain is acute. After having spent the past few days confined to bed, eating meals from trays, peeing into a bottle, he heard me bleating. He struggled out of his resting place to shuffle into the hall on his knees. Now he is glaring up at me like an irate Toulouse-Lautrec impersonator.

He is managing a tricky balancing act between fury and exasperation. He insists I have to see the doctor. How else am I going to get better? He appeals to the flickering embers of my common sense. Telling me how much I've been upsetting Mum, although I'm never aware of this because she tries masking her anguish.

Bunching my right fist I entertain the sickening impulse to spark him out. Like so many other poisonous notions, the thought materialises but evaporates.

*

The doorbell chimes. Mum announces Dr McCabe's arrival. Because I refused to visit the surgery, he has agreed to make a house call. Entering the front room to discover Dr McCabe on the settee, a folder spread over his lap, is yet another bizarre twist in my delusional existence.

He invites me to take a seat. He was in the area, so my mum's request wasn't a problem. I demand to know what he has been jotting down in his notes, although forcing this out takes an inordinate amount of time. The rest of the world is at 45 rpm but I'm stuck at 33 rpm.

Rifling through his papers seems to be a way of filling the silence. He informs me of the results of my recent blood test. Negative. This news should be a relief? I scarcely recall this blood test. When he reminds me I requested it to rule out HIV infection, I misinterpret his calming tone. Sarcasm. He's *lying*. He's just saying this so Mum won't worry. Or worry about what the neighbours might say.

I insist the neighbours are *always* talking about me. I sometimes pop a glass against the wall. Try to get the gist of the constant hubbub. I can never make it out. They disguise their poisonous conversations with code about going to the shops.

I suspect there might be a hidden passageway connecting no 3 with no 1. Dating to when these houses were first built in the 1890s. Allowing the Grahams to flit next door at any time to May Annandale's. Making it simple to ferment their plots to have us evicted.

He looks at Mum. This is the first I've realised she is sitting in on the consultation. Mum suggests I make everyone a cup of tea. So she can chat with the 'doctor.' Just milk, he says. I'm reluctant to leave them to plot.

Exiting, I close the door. Press my ear against it. McCabe murmurs about hospital treatment being no different to home treatment. Time off work. Regular medication. Rest. The decision is up to my parents. I know what he means. If I'm at home, their bugs and hidden cameras will keep me under constant surveillance. Norman Tebbit will be able to listen in.

22

Shrink

My impending visit to the Andrew Duncan Clinic. Mum: good parent. It's for your own good, son. Dr McCabe has referred you. To speak to an expert. A professional. He'll understand what you're going through.

I insist I'm not going through anything. I'll go back to bed. I've not been sleeping. Just need rest.

Dad: bad parent. Get dressed, Mark. This is ridiculous. We can't keep changing appointments. Especially since you're expected there in... Forty-three minutes.

Why should I trust the doctors at this clinic any more than Dr McCabe? *Fake.*

Dad nudges me towards my bedroom. Like a stubborn teenager, I wrench open the wardrobe. When did I last venture outside? I visualise some character in a post-apocalyptic novel. Confronting the dangers lurking beyond his bunker.

Rifling through the hangers, I select beige Chinos. Black and white striped sweatshirt. Alex and I used to joke that the only evidence of months of overtime were the tops we splashed out on during a solitary spending spree. In Next. The rest was pissed against urinals.

Alex used to call this top my Stanley Cup umpire outfit. It's been a long time since I've been slagged by mates. Now they just scorn. I wore this shirt to nightclubs. Strutted up to partying women, emboldened by alcohol. Where did that person go?

*

An attic extension is underway. Approaching the car, a hammer's rat-a-tat synchronises with my awkward gait. Goading the way my meds have stiffened my muscles. Twenty minutes later we are in the waiting area. Mum hands me a travel mag. Images of holiday resorts where the sun-dappled sea is flat as an ice rink. Smiling people draped on a golden beach where the taboo conversations will be great whites. Skin cancer.

A stout man sits opposite. I clock a tweed suit. Arthur Lowe combover. Tache. Wheezing from the exertion of strolling from his car. Suddenly, he says: Mark, isn't it? How are you?

I study him. Grant Fortune. One of my Napier lecturers. Editing and proofreading. His coincidental appearance isn't natural. More role-playing. I turn to Mum. *I'm offski.*

Tossing the magazine into Grant's lap, I spring from my seat. March for the exit. Mum heads me off. Demands I sit down again.

Like a stuck record, I whine. *Why do you think I need to see a shrink?*

She steers me back to the plastic chair. Sulking, I take in my surroundings. Become convinced I can smell fresh paint. This building suffered fire damage. Required extensive renovation. The real reason I've been tricked into coming here: they think I'm one of the arsonists.

Moments later I'm summoned to Dr Grant's office. He's a courteous, bespectacled guy. Navy tie against a denim shirt. Early 30s? But my delusions are hurtling. Whatever it might state on the nameplate on his desk, he's no more qualified than McCabe.

My last experience of fire-starting? Setting an Airfix Messerschmitt ME109 alight before launching it from my bedroom window. But that's the false memory. This interrogation is real. Grant wants a confession.

My answers range between monosyllabic mumbling and blinks. Despite this, I notice fitful biro activity. What libel is he concocting? He asks if I feel depressed. When I glower, he urges me to be honest. To try articulating the way I'm feeling. Am I anxious? Worried about anything? Do I feel down? What is making me feel down?

He invites me to consider underlying issues that could be impacting my low moods. Am I drinking a lot? Taking recreational drugs? He reacts when I mutter about magic mushrooms a couple of times as a teenager.

Do I have a regular sex life? I glare towards the blinds. He already knows that answer.

23

Poison

November 1987

The letter is signed Dr Grant, Senior House Officer of the Royal Edinburgh Hospital. I skim through it. *Depressive illness with psychomotor retardation.* Makes me think of something grinding to a halt. But the weird notions inside my head are more like a pinball machine.

Recommend amitriptyline upped to the maximum therapeutic level of 150 mg for at least six to nine months.

*

I spend hours being hypnotized by TV. During the day, quiz shows. News. After lunch, more quiz shows. More news. After tea, Brian Blessed and Hannah Gordon in *My Family and Other Animals.* Kenneth Branagh and Emma Thompson in *Fortunes of War.* Every plot drifting over my head.

The first time Mum collected my amitriptyline prescription, she read out the possible side effects. *Confusion, numbness, headaches, constipation or diarrhoea, skin rashes, swelling of the face/tongue, nausea, and unexpected weight gain/loss.* These chemicals are never going to cure me. They are having the opposite effect.

I know these capsules she presents every night on a tray, along with a mug of tea and two crackers with Edam, are a form of euthanasia.

The doctors have conspired with my parents to force-feed me poison. I'm resigned to popping each tablet into my mouth. Swallowing. Then I continue watching TV while I wait to begin feeling whatever people who have been poisoned feel. When this doesn't manifest after 20 minutes or so, I mumble goodnight. Head off to bed.

Mum is always telling me books help her deal with her own frequent bouts of sleeplessness. She loses herself in Ed McBain novels, Steve Carella chasing lowlifes across New York's 87th Precinct until she finds herself re-reading paragraphs and the novel becomes heavy as a murder weapon. So after all-too-familiar hours of tossing and turning, I claw for the light switch.

Blinking, I grope beneath my bed, retrieving the address book that has been lurking there since it was last used months before. Propping up my pillows, I open it. These names and phone numbers began accumulating as I became disinterested in playing guitar and latched onto dance music and the potential for meeting sexual partners in clubs.

Little Big Dig did reach the heady heights of that Radio 1 session. We were also featured in *The Tube* during an outside broadcast centred on the capital's Niddry Street rehearsal rooms, Jools Holland pausing outside our door while our catchiest song, 'I Get The Fear,' blared.

Our manager's then-girlfriend, Muriel had told Jools which room was ours. Maybe he forgot. He gatecrashed a neighbouring space. Lenny Helsing, formerly guitarist of one of the city's earliest punk bands, Belsen Horrors, was with bandmate Bruce, now of psychedelic garage combo The Green Telescope. The latter was rolling a large 'cigarette.' Jools ushered his camera crew away.

Muriel once listed 'I Get The Fear' in her top five songs in a fanzine interview. At the time, Holland opting not to open our door seemed another lost moment. A metaphoric blocking of a crossroads that might have led to record company recognition. Again, so irrelevant.

We were never successful enough to attract groupies. But horny singletons were to be found hanging around Lothian Road's nightspots. This address book is a window into my weekends between 1982 and whatever date equated to my last night out earlier this year. Bracketed beside the entries are the venues where we met. Some of the names conjure a face, backstories, mannerisms. Accents from Munich to Muirhouse. Many are a mystery.

The notebook describes the period when my leisure time revolved around east central Scotland's tacky nightclub scene.

Edinburgh clubs. Zenatec. Buster Brown's. Cinderella Rocke-fella's. Rumours. Gatsby's. Bobby McGee's. Outer Limits. The Hooch. Madison's. Reflections. Cat's Pyjamas. Coach trips to Bentley's and Jackie-O's in Kirkcaldy. I knew female regulars. Where they congregated. Their favourite drinks. Where they worked. Their kids' names. Their dogs' names. The teams they supported.

But for all the mirror-preening, choosing outfits, then priming myself with sufficient booze to convey the illusion of a dynamic personality, when I left a club arm-in-arm with some equally drunken female the end result was usually the dictionary definition of an anti-climax. Alcohol was a double-edged sword. Horning you up before subjecting you to 'brewer's droop.'

What impressions must've flitted through their minds when they saw me shuffling in, suit sleeves rolled up, fag in one hand, Red Stripe in the other, clichéd lines delivered in a breath reeking of lager, Marlboros, and Juicy Fruit? Their judgment would've been impaired by what Anne described as 'looking through beer goggles.'

This book is incriminating. There must be more than 50 names listed. That Gene Simmons or Robert Plant might assume this equated to five weeks rather than five years, that's scarcely any consolation.

I almost got engaged to my first serious girlfriend, Louise, our teenage crush blossoming into love against a backdrop of *Closer*, *Ju Ju*, *Talk Talk Talk*, *Seventeen Seconds* and *No*

More Heroes. But in that post-break-up vacuum, my social life became a protracted rebound. I used any excuse to drown my sorrows. Became dismissive of monogamy.

My drunken quests merely alienated these girls. Each met my brash, confident alter-ego, full of flattery. But what made the more lasting impression was the extent to which I was the opposite of that intoxicated caricature.

During sessions, I would stand women up. Ask out their best mates. Be unfaithful. Show them up in front of friends, family. Some of them might well have kept their own address books, complete with marks out of 10. I could have laughed mine off as youthful exuberance. Did Edith Piaf get it right? Regret nothing. This has become a self-help cliché. Never regret things you've done. Only the things you didn't have the courage to do.

But when news of my AIDS breaks, every single person in this book will come to despise me.

24

Finding God

I can place an exact figure on my insomnia's duration because I noticed my electronic clock when I flicked off my bedside light: 23:22. The red digits scalding my retinas now read 04:49. Five hours 27 minutes.

A thought eases through a sliver in my depressive veil. I think of those near-death experiences portrayed in medical dramas, a patient's life signal juddering. A sudden, insistent beep. I feel my pulse: the relentless tattoo that has persisted from its first instance three weeks beyond conception.

My eyes probe the shadows but with a resolve so incongruous after such a prolonged period of sinking into abject despair. Tears trickle down my face. The sensation of them tickling my features heightens the elation. I know what is happening. The thought surges through me like an electrical charge. This has affected so many people before me and although it's something I've always been as dismissive of as the existence of ghosts or the concept of a giant furnace where 'bad' people are punished for eternity, I realise it means one thing. The Holy Spirit. I've found God.

Clambering from the bed I kneel. Clasping my hands. Weeping with joy. I try articulating this euphoria, at having been lost in the darkness for so long and coming across the light at the tunnel's end. I feel the dense clouds of my desolation parting, just like the Red Sea during one of His earlier cosmic party pieces. My heartbeat thundering inside my eardrums, I remain poised, wondering what to do next.

High above Edinburgh, I hear a lone plane droning. Why should it rupture the silence right now? I acknowledge His sign by genuflecting several times.

Through my bedroom wall, Alison Graham coughs. And coughs. Her furious hacking amplifies, each phlegmy, lung-corroding outburst followed by a desperate inhalation. Like someone rescued from drowning. I hear this terrible sound coming from our neighbours every other night: the soundtrack that torments the families of workers exposed to asbestos; or in Alison's case, decades of nicotine addiction.

Medicated slumber is a respite from constant agony. I stopped playing my records loud enough for the occasional knock on the wall a long time ago. The bedroom on the other side to hers has been silent as a tomb for months. My rapturous outburst must have woken her.

I think of Michelangelo's painting on the Sistine Chapel ceiling. If the Big Yin upstairs and I did brush fingers, the moment has passed. I slink back into bed. Just myself. My free-wheeling mind. And the sound of Alison's drawn-out death.

25

Delusions

Mum has brought breakfast in bed. Placing the tray next to me, she ruffles my hair, suggests a shower and a shave after I've eaten. Everything will seem rosier after a wee dicht.

I suppose these moments of contact are the closest I'm getting to normality. Tea. Toast. Stint in the bathroom. Dining and washing are the great levellers of human society. Practised everywhere from beneath Buckingham Palace's crystal chandeliers to Death Row in Louisiana State Penitentiary.

I do devour the toast and marmalade, and if I was under close observation there would be nothing to distinguish my enthusiastic crunching from anyone else's. But when I finish and place the tray on the carpet, lifting the *Daily Express* Mum had tucked to one side, my version of reality takes over.

I used to chastise Mum, a lifelong Labour voter from Craigentinny, whose three brothers were all party members, for being an *Express* reader. I would wind her up that the term conjured someone draped in a Union Jack at Wimbledon, shooshing the protestors haranguing Buster Mottram for his National Front sympathies because it was spoiling the tennis.

I would insist most of the tabloids were owned by millionaire press barons, serving up a rancid cocktail of celebrity gossip and xenophobia, the stories spun out of all context; complex issues, literally, distilled into black and white, with any room for nuanced grey areas redacted. *The Express*, its fellow ugly sister, *The Mail*, and their delinquent siblings *The Sun* and *The Star*, were all about stoking populism, the potent agenda that guaranteed the working-class remained loyal to their country's establishment, never their own. She would shrug, admitting she did prefer the paper Dad not only bought but regularly had letters published in, *The Scotsman*. He bought *The Express* for the Rupert Bear strip cartoon. First published in 1920, the year before he was born, and in every edition ever since, Dad has grown up with Rupert.

Glancing at its front page brings fresh demoralisation. With my chemically-imbalanced mind, these neat paragraphs of typography are revealing something far more sinister than propaganda. I can relate to every bold heading because of one insidious aspect of my illness. Its solipsism.

The horrific leading story is about 11 people murdered when an IRA bomb was detonated during a Remembrance Day service in Enniskillen. There is an added poignancy because Enniskillen is where Dad lived for a while, gaining a scholarship to Portora school. My warped imagination is insisting there is more than mere coincidence involved here. This is the latest crazy event that has unfolded in the unknown, un-fathomable, haunting, and distorted world whirring around outside, with myself occupying its dark core.

The ruthless focus of my manic depression is that every newspaper headline I've been reading over the past few months, from Ian Brady announcing five more murders to Jeffrey Ryan's killing spree in the village of Hungerford, is more than just random news items. Each horrendous event forms part of an ongoing chain.

How my illness could have any connection beyond the co-incidence of timing is ludicrous, if nowhere near as deranged as 'Troubles' that have unleashed psychopaths on Irish streets, from cenotaph bombers to Shankill butchers for nearly 30 years.

Later I'm slumped on the couch while my parents chip in answering William G Stewart's questions on *Fifteen to One*. I'm not facing the TV's constant burr but gawking out the window. The sun is already sinking low over the west of the city.

I stare at this aura. Convinced there is a huge railway wagon beyond the back greens of these Shandon terraces, containing vast mirrors aiming towards that dying luminescence, captur-ing it, channelling the reflection towards the window I'm gaping through. Exposing me.

*

My folks persuaded me to accompany them to buy some seedlings. Get some fresh air into my lungs. So we're strolling around a garden centre in Balerno, below the snow-capped

Pentland Hills. I keep on firing concerned looks at Mum who has one loose button on her overcoat, hanging by threads. I know she was jostled when she went her messages yesterday. I don't want to ask her what happened. I'll just upset her more. But she was singled out for vigilante action because of me.

As it begins to grow overcast we curtail the outing. Soon we're heading back along the Lanark Road. Rain batters the car. Bouncing off the pavements. My eyes are drawn to the drops pattering the glass.

My mate Kenny once told me how his old man described the high suicide rates in UK prisons, with over 50% of the prisoners having mental health issues. This discussion went on to the Forth Road Bridge being a notorious hotspot.

I visualise the CCTV being replayed, the tape locked on fast-forward, whirring by like Rod Taylor's journey into the future in *The Time Machine*. Tankers zipping backwards and forwards to Grangemouth. *MV Gardyloo* heading out the Forth laden with tonnes of Edinburgh sewage, returning after dumping its load by St Abb's Head. Yachts flickering like erratic moths. But every so often, a minuscule splash. Like a raindrop. Or a tear. Each tiny explosion of surf the heartbreaking final moment on Earth of a lost soul, the yawning expanses of their lives' possibilities constricted into the frenetic seconds of their dive.

Then I imagine someone hitting a pause button, capturing one of these droplets at the precise moment of impact. Pressing rewind. Speeding up again. The world in reverse. The beautiful sight of all this rain soaring upwards. Back to the position where someone might have noticed them hovering then exited their car to try talking them out of it. To talk them back. To life.

As this nonsense unravels I discover I've unbuckled my seatbelt. My vision is locked on the tarmac rushing past the car. The white lines whipping underneath. I clutch the door handle. Weird, morbid curiosity more than anything self-destructive.

Dad notices the light on the dashboard. Warns me to wear my seatbelt. Glaring into the rear-view mirror, he asks Mum what those flowers were called? The white ones now stacked among the other pots in the boot?

She tells him: *Jasmines*. Even from here, in the back, I can smell their honey-like aroma. It makes my stomach turn.

26

02

Time passes at a uniform rate, its passage signified by segments allocated by ancient mathematicians according to periods of sunlight and shadow. We can approximate the length of a second, sometimes by prefacing it with three syllables. *One Mississippi. Two Mississippi...* Ironic. In a Mississippi penitentiary, human life is sometimes distilled into crucial minutes and seconds in the lethal injection room, except the officials administering the sodium thiopental, pancuronium bromide, and potassium chloride don't count using their State. They'll refer to digital countdowns before pronouncing death.

I feel my consciousness drifting. Aimless. A marooned raft. What does the clock say? How long have I been lying in this particular position? What was that noise out in the back green? The wind? A fox?

I dwell on everything worrying me. Fraying my nerves. Except worrying should be reserved for identifiable subjects.

Family. Money. Relationships. Health. Politics. Addictions. None of these is the source of my worries. My mind has been infected with arrant nonsense.

However my worries might have originated somewhere on Planet Earth, they have long since broken free of their moorings in the innermost recesses of my imagination. Reaching a point where they are no longer worries at all because worries can always be contextualised with counter-arguments. With sanity. My worries are now a horrid, all-encompassing cloud. Dense. Black. Pitiless. Almost a tangible thing contaminating every pore of my being.

If there is a sea-bed beneath the sludge at the base of the Marianna Trench of my wretchedness, this is where my consciousness now lurks. Within the impenetrable fog stifling my former intellect.

Pawing into the darkness, I reach for the half-pint tumbler perched next to my bed. Tip the water over the carpet. Grasping it by the handle I aim for the wall. Intending to shatter it, then plunge the shards deep into my skin. Instead of cutting across you hack down. Elbow to the hand. I recall that enlightening factoid from drunken pub chat.

Except seconds pass, until the glass becomes a dead weight in my hand. Allowing it to slip through my fingers into the puddle, I stare into the void. My unravelling sanity concocts an even more insane twist.

Every thought driven by anxiety and crashed self-esteem, I reiterate to myself how worthless I feel. And there's only one way to stop all this horrible, demeaning, self-loathing.

After my failure with the glass, I picture the U-Boat from *Das Boot*, a TV drama I was hooked on when I was capable of connecting with anything. I imagine being a sailor in that metal capsule. Languishing in the void above the silt on the seabed. Cowering from depth charges. Hull ruptured. A survivor hemmed into a last pocket of air. When all the oxygen is used it will be a case of expiring. A pale light, getting dimmer. Dimmer. Fizzling into darkness.

I read drowning was peaceful. Painless. People fortunate enough to be fished from water spoke of having been enveloped by an incredible sense of calm. So. I decide I'll just stop breathing. Until the light fades. Goes out. Taking a deep breath, I hold onto it.

Vague notions slither around my fucked-up perception. Visions of those drowners, fading into the ocean depths. Back into the cradle of life.

Counting the seconds. One Mississippi to 60 Mississippi. Pain begins emanating from my rib-cage. 75. This spreads further. Seeping to my throat. 90 Mississippi. Centres on my Adam's apple. 100 Mississippi. Tiny lights spark behind my eyelids. 105 Mississippi. The longer I hold my breath the more I become aware of myself. I feel nauseous. My throat aches and further pinpoints of agony erupt throughout my body: forehead, temples, crotch. 110 Mississippi. This is no gentle slipping away.

My mind may have wandered but my body is disturbed by this violation. A pulse tattoos at my neck. 120 Mississippi. Becomes an insistent rhythm, a trapped submariner using his final breaths to drum a spanner against his stricken vessel's hull. My bloodstream craves oxygen. There is nothing relaxed or effortless about this. 125 Missippi. My lungs give an involuntary spasm. Snatch a breath. Air flows into my lungs. I prevent the next breath, count to 60 Missppi... Beyond... Near 120 Mippi. Involuntarily inhaling again. Back to zero.

No idea how long I continue this. Delusional as I am, I can accept this form of self-harm is impossible.

27

Sectioned

As children, Anne and I grew to fear trips to our dentist, Dr Wise, with his balding white hair and pronounced German accent. The drilling equipment he applied when inflicting eye-watering fillings without any painkilling jags seemed rudimentary. Coupled with that accent, it was so easy for us to imagine being in the clutches of a Nazi fugitive, like Laurence Olivier's character in *Marathon Man*. Dentistry as torture. In truth, Mum told us his family fled Germany three decades earlier, before the evil storm. Dr Wise was Jewish. Not only that, his granddaughter has special needs; had she lived under the Third Reich she would have been euthanised.

But I'm recalling one occasion when I was anaesthetised before having four teeth extracted. I remember being led from his surgery, stumbling like a newborn foal. Consciousness seeping back in fits and starts, I loved the dreamy sensation.

Couldn't stop sniggering. Imagined how wonderful it would be to feel this dizzy all the time.

There's a rising sense of alarm. Being smothered by an anaesthetist's rubber mask for minutes of trippy dreams then their giddy aftermath was one thing. This new reality is off the scale.

I'm inside a bare room. On a single bed. Draped in a thin polyester blanket. I'm in pyjamas. I've no recollection of changing into them. Like so many hazy Sundays where the night before culminated in an alcoholic void, I try piecing events together.

The memories are cartoon-like. I feel a narcotic edge. As if I'm emerging from a stupor after being spiked. There was an ambulance. This brings a pang of alarm that spurs sobriety. I've no idea who brought me into this bedroom. But now I remember Mum being led in by some stranger. She was wearing a yellow raincoat and dabbing her eyes with the hankie she always scrunches under her wrist.

The background noise is indistinct. A TV. Footfall. Voices ranging from muted conversation to someone continually shouting what sounds like *Mum!* I focus on the frost-caked window beyond a grille. Heavy footfall. Keys jangle. A door slams. This panics me with the notion I'm in prison.

A man enters. Sits on the one chair facing the bed. Wearing a white shirt and tie, he is stocky, with round glasses that exaggerate what I perceive to be Japanese features. My warped perception makes me think of a stereotypical camp guard in a

Commando comic. But he fixes me with a smile before refer-ring to a notebook.

He asks if know where I am. I just stare. He tells me I was agitated. Disturbed. He refers to my *episode*. My mother phoned an ambulance. I was given tranquillizers. Now I'm in hospital.

My reaction is to gawk. Open-mouthed as a caveman wit-nessing fire. He writes something. I close my eyes.

*

The timebomb has ignited. For months I've been a slave to par-anoia, delusion, insomnia, self-loathing – and they're just four of the stampede of horsemen of the bipolar apocalypse. Now I'm in limbo, comfortably numbed by pills. The GP-prescribed meds I've been guzzling might as well have been Revels. My medication has been taken to a whole new level. Rather than being relaxed, this is more like a chemical exorcism.

*

I'm led into a room where I'm confronted by two women. Two males. I've no idea who they are. Doctors? Detectives? The older female is explaining something.

One symptom of my illness concerns doppelgangers. As soon as I meet someone for the first time, my fertile imagina-tion conjures their closest lookalike from the people I already know. This inexplicable phenomenon stokes my paranoia. Makes me assume their appearance is no coincidence.

This woman is the double of a neighbour, Cathy Sheen. She even *sounds* like Cathy. As she informs me I'm being formally sectioned, I ask if she's related to Cathy Sheen. Commenting I'm mistaking her for someone else, she proceeds.

Later, I'll discover this moment is the cornerstone of mental health care. The section is the actual legislation underlying the clichéd statement of someone becoming 'certifiable'. Right now, her words wash over me.

You need to understand what we mean when we say you're being sectioned, that is, admitted to hospital under section three of the Mental Health (Scotland) Act of 1984. When you're sectioned it sets in motion a train of events. We'll start addressing the problems you've been facing, Mark, because at least three health professionals, and your parents, feel you're no longer fit enough to ask for help yourself. Sometimes patients are not even aware they're ill. Others have reached a stage where their illness has made them a threat to themselves or others. This section... you could say it strips away many of the rights we all enjoy as a functioning members of society... but it's only to allow your rehabilitation to become the overriding concern. We'll have twenty-eight days to assess you, Mark. Also, it's now illegal for you to vote, leave the country, or apply for a passport.

I nod at this person who has been designated to confront me because she resembles a woman who lives across the street. Cathy's double might as well have been hypothesising about the mysterious dark matter forming 85% of the universe.

28

False Imprisonment

Over the following days, my mental confusion persists, stoked by unfamiliar surroundings, lengthy periods of solitude, and the persistent impression everyone is staring at me. This ward is locked. Whenever I hear a grating key as a nurse changes shift I imagine rushing the gap. Will alarms ring throughout the hospital? Will it be like *One Flew Over The Cuckoo's Nest*: a frantic chase terminated by a rugby tackle and a needle?

My swirling anxieties do have moments of lucidity. I peer at the photo by my bedside. Mum, Dad, and Anne, beaming at a Chinese banquet. Celebrating Anne's birthday almost a year ago, I had no way of knowing the nightmare ahead. But I can accept how fortunate I am to have this loving family.

*

A grey-bearded bloke shambles into the dorm during the night in a stained overcoat, enveloped by a fug of alcohol and street grime. He collapses onto a spare bed without removing his boots. Spends the night snoring. Farting. Grumbling in his troubled sleep. Everywhere he visits in his dreams it sounds as if he always ends up snarling while being ejected. Mental illness and homelessness. Vicious circle.

*

Developing perspective, I can see myself surrounded by patients who seem at much more extreme points of the manic scale. Most seem content to take root in the lounge. If you do amble through to your bed and stretch out, the nurses follow you. Implore you to get up. Daytime snoozing is discouraged because it might hinder a good night's sleep: an important aspect of recovery.

Some patients have ants in their pants. Swarms of them. Fraser is a wiry teenager with hair that appears to have been combed with barbed wire. He scuffs along the corridor in odd socks, smokes fags right into the filter. Another young guy, Ritchie, wears a biker jacket like a layer of skin. After lights out he crashes out on his bed, still wearing that jacket.

Ritchie marches in and out of rooms, laser-eyed, nostrils flaring. I nickname him Fonz, although he's more like a switchblade-wielding greaser from *Rumblefish* than the cuddly rogue from *Happy Days*. Like Siamese fish, Fraser and Ritchie sometimes launch punches at each other and have to be separated by staff.

There's one patient I only see being steering into the canteen in a wheelchair, where his meals are spooned in by a nurse while he gapes beyond the barred windows.

A more constant presence is Martha, a white-haired woman who shuffles into the lounge or along the corridor in pink slippers. Her doppelganger is my childhood piano teacher, Mrs Stevenson, a quiet, churchy woman who would jam Anne and my fingers into the keyboard when our lack of weekly practice translated into repeated bum notes. Except Martha's vocabulary is an unrelenting stream of muttered curses against her fellow patients, the medical staff, and God. Often she'll conclude one of her rants by lifting her nightdress to reveal her preference for going commando.

The more I settle into my new lifestyle, one chink of reason begins encroaching through my depressive fog, a notion that grows in momentum. I come to a conclusion. This has all been a terrible mistake. I'm not supposed to be here at all. No way. This seems as irrefutable as the knowledge the sun is sinking in the direction of Craiglockhart Hill each afternoon.

So I decide I'll demand someone lets me out through that locked door. I stop the nearest nurse. Magnus, according to his badge. Magnus smiles as I approach, then gazes at the floor while I try explaining. This is difficult. I've spent so long lost inside interior monologues that expressing them seems impossible.

Mumbling about miscarriages of justice, I stab a finger to-wards the nearest window. Notice how this gesture exposes my shaking arm. Magnus clocks that. Informs me I look a bit more agitated than usual today. This pumps up my bit of agitation ten-fold.

If I don't make myself clear I might have to bolt for the door. Then I consider the rugby-tackling. The needle preceding a nausea-inducing anaesthetic. I announce I need to go. Now. He assumes I'm referring to the toilet. His voice drops into a soothing whisper that makes me feel five again, on the first day of primary one, lurking terrified in the playground. In my mind, I regress, shrinking in height to cower beneath this scary adult. I tell him he isn't understanding. Four-syllables. Progress.

The charge nurse strides by. Grey-haired with a dark moustache, he reminds me of the 1970s TV detective *McCloud* although his harsh voice isn't New Mexican. It's somewhere north of the Forth Bridge on 30-a-day. He tells Magnus he'll deal with me. Invites me into his office.

I take in his family photo centred on the desk. He asks me to take a seat. As I sit, he shuffles papers out the way, perches his backside on the edge of the desk.

He wants me to explain my predicament. Delves into his jacket, tugs out a 20-pack of B&H. Flipping the lid he offers one. I pluck it out, struggling with my shakes, then lean forward to accept his lighter. Taking a long drag I wince. This seems akin to inhaling noxious fumes.

As my mind drifts to mustard gas wafting over the Somme mud, smoke splutters from my nose and mouth. My coughing fit persists until I can feel my cheeks flaring. Catching my beetroot-like reflection in the portrait's glass, I jack-knife the full-length snout into an overflowing ashtray on the desk. Mutter, I stopped smoking weeks ago.

He arches his eyebrows, quipping that whatever else is eating me, at least it won't be cancer. But he cuts his chuckle short, folding his arms. Inside I am brimming with a rant against the injustice of finding myself incarcerated in a psychiatric hospital, ordered to take pills at regular intervals, having to shave and shower while a nurse attends because I'm under 'close observation.' Why do I need to be under close observation? I sense eyes on me all the time. I feel as outraged as some lifer who knows the real culprit's identity.

But my turmoil remains internal. A notion flits into my head. Raising my hands, I improvise sign language. He watches my absurd display for the time it takes my wrists to grow tired. As a charge nurse in a locked psychiatric ward, there will be few manifestations of mental instability he hasn't clapped his world-weary eyes on. Maybe there's a medical expression for pretend tic-tac?

He marches beyond me. Holds the door open. Whatever empathy he felt has been quashed. Was my latest performance enough to merit a paragraph in my case notes or an irritation? I make straight to my bedroom to rummage for a Juicy Fruit.

29

Blank

In the visitors' room. A nurse sits opposite. 'Shona McDougall' on her badge. Shona has a clipboard over her lap, a sheet of lined A4 bulldog-clipped to it. She seems a few years younger than me. She breaks the awkward silence by asking if I'm aware why I'm in hospital. She waits. I watch her expression altering from patience to concern. Eyebrows arching.

She repeats the question. When I remain mute, she runs through the events that have led to me being sectioned. It sounds like the plot of a David Cronenberg film. I was self-harming. Headbutting my bedroom wall. Grappling with my parents who resorted to phoning 999 and summoning an ambulance. Because I was being violent, a police escort was also despatched. I was taken to the Royal Infirmary, to Casualty. After refusing to exit the ambulance, I was taken here to the Royal Edinburgh Hospital. I'm in the Intensive Psychiatric Care Unit.

I notice an air-conditioning grille above her head. Do I hear an imperceptible hiss? The less I pay attention to her, the more I can sense the air being drained. I stare at this grille continuing to suck oxygen from the atmosphere. At what point will we start gasping for breath? My pulse patters. Mouth feels parched. When she applies her biro to the page, her movements appear sluggish. Growing more laboured. Time is slowing. An effect of oxygen deprivation. Murmuring something, she stands and opens the door. Leaves. I gasp as the cool air rushes back.

*

Leigh is a slight, pretty nurse, blue eyes twinkling beneath a sleek, dark brown bob. Although all the girls in my life are exes, Leigh could be a younger sister of my most recent one, Helen. Helen and I got together in Buster Browns and dated during the weeks before my paranoid agoraphobia outweighed my libido.

Leigh leads a band of us out of the ward and on a short jaunt to a kitchen block. After melding various ingredients together, snowstorms of flour end up over worktops, floor, patients. Her admonishing us like kids reinforces my sense of having regressed to childhood. I doubt if anyone will have the bottle to sample the mysterious mixture she slides into the oven.

30

Teenage Rampage

We are seated around a long table. Shona hands out sheets of A3 paper. Paint palettes. Jars of water. Brushes. We've to paint something. *Anything.* Find our inner Picasso. Another patient, Don whistles the viewers' gallery theme from *Vision On.* Focusing on the blank canvas, I feel a sliver of a grin.

Dipping my brush into the paint, I smear the paper with generous brushstrokes. Emerald green. The colour of the football scarf once pinned to my headboard, programmes that had pride of place on the bedroom wall I targeted with my forehead days before.

Pretending to admire my crude artwork, Shona observes there's a Hibernian fan at the table. Muted approval or groans.

*

After tea I'm on my bed, gawking into the ceiling. Movement in the corner of my eye. Ritchie hovers by the doorway. Paces over to where Fraser is slumbering. Grasps his hair. Shrugging him off, Fraser launches his covers over him like a gladiator's net. He leaps onto the writhing shape. Digging his hands in. Seizing Ritchie's head. Thumping it into the floor. Seconds later, two male nurses rush in. Haul them apart. Ritchie protests his innocence while being frogmarched out of the dorm. While Fraser looks on, rubbing his even more dishevelled hair, a nurse heaves his bedclothes back into place. Catching my gaze, he thanks me for not jumping in.

*

Don strolls over. Mentioning the art therapy, he hands me a hardback. *100 Years of Hibs* by Gerry Docherty and Phil Thomson, with a forward by Sir Matt Busby. On the cover, Joe Harper slots the ball past Stuart Kennedy of Rangers.

In a monotone laden with meds, he talks about the goalie, Jim Herriot. Started his working life as a brickie. Went on to win the League Cup. Two Dryburgh Cups. Eight Scotland caps. Used to put boot polish around his eyes to deflect the glare from headlights, made him look like a fucking panda. Played for the Pars, then went to Birmingham. During one match, a spectator called James Wight noticed his name in the programme. James became a vet in Yorkshire. Wrote books about being a vet. Used the name, James Herriot.

I nod at that, appreciating the anecdotes in this volatile ward. It also adds fuel to the emotions kindled earlier. Before my illness, when I could have leisure interests, I was obsessive about music far more than sport. And while most wee boys inherit their football teams from dads, stepdads, or older siblings, Dad detested sport. Except for snooker. But his Irish roots and the sentimental songs he loved listening to as an accompaniment to his Carlsberg Specials meant I chose Hibs as my team.

Flicking through the book, memories flood back. Season 1973-1974. My first as a spectator. Christmas was marked by a race to top the charts between Slade's 'Merry Christmas' and Wizzard's 'I Wish It Could Be Christmas Everyday.' Two songs destined to festive immortality. Noddy Holder's band won the Black Country duel.

On Christmas morning, I tore one parcel open. A scarf. Green and white chevrons. The previous January the family enjoyed our traditional New Year's dinner at my Uncle David and Auntie Mary's in Willowbrae. My uncle and cousin Ross were Jambos; my uncle, who ended up lecturing in computer science at Heriot-Watt, used to travel to away games. Bashing a tambourine. I recall his increasing despair at the news filtering over the radio. Although Hibs were away in the Ne'er Day derby we were five-nil up by half-time, adding two more before the final whistle.

I picture that scarf pinned to my bedroom wall, alongside mementoes handed in by Billy Annandale next door. Programmes. Barcelona, Fairs Cup quarter-final, February 1961. Sporting Lisbon, Cup Winners Cup, July 1972, an encounter the home team won 6-1. Poland's Gornik Zabrze, friendly, December 1969. Centremost the *Evening News* souvenir poster celebrating our 1972 League Cup triumph over Celtic.

Childhood heroes pop into my mind: Alex Cropley, Alan Gordon, Pat Stanton, Jimmy O'Rourke, Eric Schaedler, Jim

Herriot, Alex Edwards, Jim Black, Des Bremner, Arthur Duncan, John Blackley, John Brownlie. Turnbull's Tornadoes.

Further memories stir. The week before, I spent the evening at a mate's at the top end of my street. Craig, also in my primary class, had a maroon scarf draped over his headboard. We would sketch our teams' goals the previous weekend. Complete with arrows showing the direction of crosses and shots. As I was heading home, a mob of youths tore past like stampeding horses, platform soles clattering.

Amongst them, I recognised the lads who hung around outside the launderette on Ashley Terrace in their Bay City Roller high waisters, responsible for spraypainting Young Shandon Terror on the parkie's hut in Harrison Park.

Mum crossed swords with the YST once, returning from the Dominion after taking Anne and me to see *What's Up Doc?* Plastic bags stuffed with garden refuge were stacked outside the Ettrick Hotel, which the lads were ripping open with Stanley knives. Ordering us to walk ahead, Mum strode over and demanded they stop. They were immature enough to giggle, then take to their heels, swinging their arms, crying, *Let's play aeroplanes!*

Like neighbourhood gangs across Edinburgh, they would merge into the largest local clan for tear ups. For Shandon's aspiring terracing thugs, this meant Gorgie Jungle. I watched them squeezing through the gap in the fence above the steep embankment leading down to the railway, prised apart by generations of kids.

My pals and I used to relish weekend escapes into that dangerous playground of railway tracks, bridges, tunnels and marshalling yards patrolled by irate men in bright overalls. Preparing to confront imagined versions of German or Japanese patrols. Growing up in the 1960s, the war was only a couple of decades ago. Many of the middle-aged men in our community would have served.

These lads squirming through the fencing were doing what gangs had done for generations, 'playing' at war. Possibly heading for a pre-arranged clash with youths from beyond the Meggetland playing fields. Most likely their Oxgangs counterparts. Bar-Ox.

Just before the last youth writhed through, he cast a furtive glance over his shoulder. Perhaps wondering if his gang had been noticed. One reason for such a public display of mob rule was the thrill of being the centre of attention. Five years later I would experience the same buzz each time a bunch of us clambered aboard a bus in our punk DMs and gaudy badges. He had to make do with a gawking 11-year-old in a parka, and Mrs Geppie from number 51 tugging her blind poodle.

His russet hair, reaching to his denim collar, spiked on top, reminded me of Bowie on the cover of *Alladin Sane*, the stylistic point of origin for thousands of facsimiles across the country. *He's outrageous, he screams and he bawls.* I imagined following, becoming swept up in their mad rampage. Instead, I scuffed home to finish colouring in my cartoon summary of Hibs 3-1 victory over St Johnstone.

Whether it's the sense of emerging from a lengthy self-exile, or the ever-present fag stench in this ward – an aroma I'll forever associate with my first ventures to Easter Road – other recollections from that era are vivid.

March 9th 1974. Scottish Cup, 5th round. Hibs v. Dundee. After Dad paid us in through the father and son turnstile, I mounted the steps, anticipation rising as the cauldron of noise from the other side carried. At the summit, I caught my breath at the sight of the arena sprawling before me. I'd never been amongst so many other people. Thousands. *Tens* of thousands. (The *Evening News* later stated 28,236.)

The atmosphere was electric, the tannoy blasting 'Tigerfeet' by Mud. 'Radar Love' by Golden Earring. 'Street Life' by Roxy Music. Songs I'd recorded on my portable cassette player, its microphone pointing at the transistor radio to capture tinny versions of the swaggering glam rock. But the song that encapsulated the glamour of being on the cusp of your teens was the one that rang through my head when I remembered YST haring along the road. 'The Jean Genie.'

On *Top of the Pops* the glam rockers all wore feather cuts. Just like so many of the older teenagers eyeing me up as I weaved through the throng. Many were smoking. Sipping beer cans. Slugging half-bottles. Never knotted to their necks, scarves were strapped to wrists or worn as makeshift belts around high-waisted bags.

There was an air of expectancy about the cup tie. Also tension. Teenage gangs were rife. Along with Gorgie Jungle and Bar-Ox, there were Tollcross Rebels. Clerrie Jungle. Porty Rebels. Lochend Shamrock. Granton Young People. Maggie Youth Team. Young Leith Team. Young Niddrie Terror. They were supposed to communicate with hand signals, like tic-tac. YNT used their pinkies for their sign. Gorgie Jungle a fist, pinkie and forefinger outstretched. Except the latter sign would only flash on these terraces if Hearts were the opposition. Away from here many of these lads would resort to their local street mob, Saturday unity lapsing into neighbourhood rivalries.

There were also rumours of gangs from Dundee lurking in the Dunbar End. With no segregation, there were just as many surly youths wearing dark blue. Chanting. Clapping. Fist-pumping. There was a pervading sense the throng could part at any moment while yobs would identify targets according to their colours, swing punches, launch stack-heeled shoes.

I scampered to the front leaving dad and his friend, Derek amongst drunkenly aggressive Dundonians. Not young hooligans. Grown men and women surrounded by bulging carry-out bags. Dad later told Mum he'd never heard so much swearing, especially from the dark-blue bedecked women. At one point one of the latter squatted and tried pissing into an empty beer can.

Flicking through this book I come across a close-up of the main terracing from what could well have been that tie. It had been a see-sawing encounter. The Dees opened the scoring. Alan Gordon equalised. Dundee took the lead again. Gordon completed a hat-trick to give us a 3-2 lead. They pulled one back to secure a replay at Dens Park nine days later which they won 3-0.

I scan the crowd on the long-vanished main terracing. Frozen in monochrome, a sea of feather-cuts, parkas, and wide lapels. I discover a man in his early 50s with Eric Morecambe's glasses and combover, smoking a cigar. Surrounded by faces reacting with joy and consternation to events on the pitch, he seems a lone figure, press-ganged into attendance, rooted to his watch.

31

Iggy Pop

I spend most of my time in the lounge, passive smoking hundreds of cigarettes. Beyond a galaxy of fag burns on the carpet tiles, the room's focal point is the TV. After the evening meal, chairs are arranged in rows before this altar. Although I've watched for hours, news reports and drama plots just wash over me, like the shimmering backdrop beyond a goldfish bowl.

Sportscene does stand out on what must be Saturday. I overhear a nurse chatting during the highlights of Celtic's 4-0 trouncing of Dunfermline. He was there, in the Jungle. Andy Walker showing how to take penalties. Twice. Frank McAvennie scoring his fifth since joining from West Ham in October. He mentions McAvennie being the club's record signing. Three-quarters of a million. Souness approached him at last year's World Cup in Mexico. Wanted him to be Rangers first Catholic signing to signal his bold new direction.

Obviously, Macca knocked the fucking Huns back. Signing a token Uncle Tam's not going to stop the legions singing The Sash.

Later, a nurse plonks himself down. Winks at me. Jangles his keys. All the staff carry keychains for this locked ward. But his subtle clinking is code. This is how the staff communicate without any of us understanding. I watch him swap the bunch of keys to his other hand. When his keys are delved into a pocket, it's the cue for another nurse to stand up. Yawn and stretch. Exit.

What messages are being relayed? The longer they keep me trapped in here, the more chance of me cracking their code.

*

The chairs have been stacked against the walls. A teenage girl places a bulky cassette player onto the carpet. Smiles at the nine patients, introduces herself as Susan, an occupational therapist. For this morning's keep-fit session we've to follow her movements and she'll allow us plenty of opportunities for breathers. She pokes a button. I recognise Olivia Newton-John's 'Physical.'

I can't remember when I last paid attention to music. A chasm opened during the summer. After buying albums and singles, playing in bands that performed gigs, recorded demos and albums, even being broadcast on Radio 1 and Radio Forth, my interest waned like a dying bulb. Despite an enthusiasm coursing throughout my teens and into my 20s, I became more comfortable with silence. It dawns on me this cheesy song, with its dance-lite beat, insipid lyrics but catchy melodies, is the first time I've *listened* to music for months.

Olivia's implores that there's nothing left to talk about unless it's done horizontally. Lust is such a prevailing undercurrent of pop music yet individual songs have always been vilified by the Mary Whitehouses of this world. Typified by the BBC banning Gang of Four's *rubbers you hide*, Frankie Goes To Hollywood when Holly Johnson sang about avoiding coming, and OMD's 'Enola Gay' for glorifying homosexuality.

While the eradication of sexual desire from my own radar has been an obvious symptom of my depression, I now recall how Anne used to say one ex, Louise reminded her of Olivia Newton-John, especially when she dyed her hair peroxide. That notion does spark long-suppressed emotions. Puts me in mind of another song entitled 'Physical' that was way more intense. By Adam and the Ants.

Long before Adam's chart-topping, swashbuckling shtick, sporting the hussar tunic worn by David Hemmings in *The Charge of the Light Brigade*, he was reviled by the music press. Prompted to write 'Press Darlings' in reply. He was supposed to be a punk but refused to tow what had become the conformist, anti-establishment line. Ignoring anarchy, fascism and boredom, his songs celebrated bondage, sadomasochism, dominance and submission. Ant music for sex people.

I snigger at everyone following Susan's lead. Gyrating from side to side. Stretching. Straining to touch toes. Groaning at the unfamiliar muscle strains. Hesitant about participating, I step forward. Now we're marching on the spot. I stomp my feet up and down.

You can't help but laugh at the incongruous way we express our love of music by dancing. Moving to the beat. From Polynesian villages to Detroit house clubs to a locked psychiatric unit, the way music inspires self-expression with synchronised movement is one of the most wonderful human instincts.

In the doorway, I spot two nuns nodding to the beat. I've no idea how often nuns visit the ward, but one patient has RFC inked into his neck. I wait for the inevitable reaction as he snaps out of exercising to utter something poisonous. He's too busy jogging on the spot.

The more immediate concern for Susan is Martha, who has materialised behind the nuns in her dressing-gown. Her agitated speech rises above the music. Appreciating her furious four-letter outbursts against God would faze the most dutiful of his servants, a nurse ushers her away.

I feel a weird irony performing star jumps in front of nuns, stretching my limbs like St Andrew's crucifixion. When Susan tells us to take five, a tall bloke approaches me. Someone new to the ward. A nurse or a fresh patient? He answers this by asking if I think I'm Jesus Christ. When I tell him I'm many things, but *not* the Messiah, he pats my shoulder. Tells me this is just as well. Because *he's* Jesus Christ.

A balding guy in a shapeless cardigan overhears. Demands to know if my inquisitor just claimed to be Jesus. When this is affirmed, he announces he is God. The lad shakes his hand with exuberance. *Hiya, Dad!*

We resume jumping on the spot. Closing my eyes, I'm reminded of pogoing. Taken back to my youth.

Clouds is rammed with tousle-haired kids. Clothes spray-painted. Festooned with pins and chains. My white T-shirt, the one I wore to PE last year, marker-penned with band names.

BUZZCOCKS. DEAD BOYS. THE CORTINAS. JOHNNY THUNDERS AND THE HEARTBREAKERS. EATER. MENACE. CRISIS. ATV. ULTRAVOX! THE SAINTS. WIRE. THE FREEZE. SCARS. GEN X. CHELSEA. THE CLASH. 999.

The heat has plastered its cotton to my skin. My Harrington is tied around my waist, revealing ANTZ: ANTMUSIC FOR SEXPEOPLE daubed across my shoulder blades. The Ants' London gigs draw cult followers wearing fetish gear, PVC masks, reflecting their song titles: 'Beat My Guest,' 'Whip in My Valise,' 'Rubber People.' Does fantasising about Servalan from *Blake's 7* in her black leather uniforms make me a sex person?

The lights cut. A pregnant pause. Everyone craning towards the stage. Before me, two punkettes, brunette and peroxide blonde. Arms linked. Perfume potent, an intoxicating aphrodisiac. Hair sculpted with egg whites into Statue of Liberty spikes, like Adam Ant's onetime collaborator and occasional backing singer, Jordan. The blonde in a torn blouse. The brunette a fishnet vest revealing her bra. Homage to The Slits.

Unlike the rock bands I've seen with my schoolmate Kenny, Blue Oyster Cult and Judas Priest, where the audiences were overwhelmingly denim-clad lads, there are hordes of female fans in this seething mass. Ensuring a frisson of sexual tension courses through this thrilling new music scene.

Thinking of Kenny makes me chuckle. We have frequent debates about the merits of this *new wave* compared to the *boring old farts* he still champions. The last time he was round, we arsed a half-bottle of Smirnoff. In the finest spirit of 'if you can't beat them, join them,' he was bouncing around my bedroom to The Vibrators' live B-side, Stiff Little Fingers.

Prescient. A roar from the front, gathering momentum until everyone is cheering, whistling. The stage lights ignite, revealing Stiff Little Fingers. In a gruff Belfast brogue encapsulating fury at the decades of mindless sectarian violence instigated by the partitioning of their homeland, Jake Burns barks about a suspect device that has left two thousand dead.

They're *so* fast. I throw myself into the melee, leaping up and down, the pricks near the front launching salvos of spit. Through the confusion, I glimpse one of the mates I came in with but lost, Ross. He started a band last year. The Accidents. Earlier they touched base with the lad who's going to be their new guitarist, Graham. He's a chef in Goldbergs. His hair is dyed green. I clock several green barnets bouncing in the middle of all this. Everyone is leaping up and down and stumbling and struggling back up and howling the words and although I've got school in the morning I don't care. An uncertain future might be yawning before me but there's nothing beyond this moment, and the music's passion and energy.

Susan presses 'stop.' Like everyone else I'm breathless, heart thumping. I'm visualising the flat-line of my depression starting to pulse again. Tightening my fists, I savour this heartbeat. My life's relentless drum. I imagine this as the rhythm of so many songs I've long forgotten; the records and tapes that have been gathering dust in my bedroom for months.

I need to listen to them again. *All* of them. Every single and flip side. Every album track, from polished studio cuts to the raw recordings capturing the essence of live performances. Somewhere inside there's still the essence of a naïve 16-year-old punk. A disciple of Iggy Pop. Lusting for life.

32

Visitors

Throughout the wallowing seas of my depression, my appetite has remained an island of sanity. I relish the meals I ticked on menu cards the day before. Other patients are not as fortunate as me and have to be cajoled into eating. Or just won't show. So there are always unclaimed trays.

Today I'm tucking into a strawberry trifle, a poor imitation of the ones I'm used to. Mum works as a cook in a home for retired nurses in Kingsknowe. At home we have our taste buds spoiled. But it's appetising enough.

I identify this is Wednesday. Two nurses are predicting how many goals Lineker will score for Barcelona against some Albanian side in the UEFA Cup. A glimpse of a world so distant it's like overhearing a conversation between Mission Control and astronauts.

After the meal, I shuffle back to the dorm. I flick through the Hibs book. Magnus approaches. Tells me my family is here. I follow him along the corridor. Fraser is hovering by the visitor room, glaring at the unrecognised faces. When I get to the window I see Mum, Dad, and Anne. If my bloodstream wasn't so pumped with sedatives I would've been euphoric.

After the distraction of Martha demanding to know who the fuck these cunts are, Magnus ushering her away while explaining they're Mark's family, I enter. Close the door. I clutch Mum the longest. Burying my face in her shoulder. Inhaling her perfume. The moment distills a hundred previous experiences when I sought refuge after scraping my knees playing in the street, or having been clouted by a bigger lad. Now I have to bend down.

Dad keeps patting my shoulder while Anne strokes my sleeve. Mum mentions talking to a Dr Gilchrist who I assume is an older guy I've noticed striding up and down the ward, files tucked under his arm. He told her he was satisfied with how I'm responding to my course of drugs. It dawns on me Dr Gilchrist and Dr McCabe from my own surgery *are* doctors. Not inquisitors. Or hooligans.

I mutter I'm feeling better. Ask how they're all doing. Anne describes going to see a Woody Allen double bill at The Filmhouse with her best friend, Lesley. *Hannah and Her Sisters* and *Manhattan*. She adds Lesley is going to make up a Stranglers compilation on cassette for me to listen to. She's asked when she can visit. Mum chips in that cousin John was on the phone. Another Stranglers connection. John and I were excitable school kids when we first saw them eight years ago, headlining the Loch Lomond Festival, their performance culminating in 'Down in the Sewer' beneath a firework display. Earlier that day we had our photo taken with Nicky Garrett, guitarist of one of the support acts, U.K. Subs. Remembering myself in a black and mauve mohair jumper, beaming next to Nicky with striped hair brings a flicker of a smile.

Mum tells me about Grannie. Last year, she broke her hip after slipping on black ice in Craigentinny. But when she received the news about her grandson, the first thing she did was pop over to those same shops to buy flowers for Mum and a bottle of whisky for Dad. Then she walked all the way to Kemp's Corner to get the bus across town.

Fraser marches by. He seems furious these newcomers are encroaching on his space. But I've come to recognise that's down to his meds. His expression was just as intense when he tucked into his cereal this morning.

We exchange small talk for about 20 minutes. When the time comes to depart, I chum them to the door. A nurse draws out his chained keys to lock it behind them. I watch them go, listening to Mum's clicking heels fading.

I head to the TV lounge. Immerse myself in the screen, trying to forget what a wrench it was not to just walk out with them. A film unfolds before me. I concentrate on the impossibility of catching up with the storyline through a medicated haze and an unwillingness to engage with the other viewers.

When the credits roll a nurse delivers supper: a large tray bearing plates piled high with bread and jam pieces. There are pots of tea. A cup is poured for me. I take a piece over to my chair, excess raspberry jam trickling around my wrist. I lick my skin, relishing the bittersweet taste. Just like I did when I was exercising here the other day, I get the feeling that for the first time in a long, dark period, things may be looking up.

33

John Peel

Just as I'm settling to gawk at daytime TV, a nurse, Duncan taps my shoulder. He wonders how I'm feeling. Okay, I say, shrugging. Nodding, he informs me I'm getting transferred to Ward 5 today. My expression must betray alarm, but he assures me this development is nothing to worry about.

He explains Ward 5 is an *open* ward. I'll be allowed to pop out to the shops, to Morningside Library. Maybe a trip up to the Dominion now and again. He was there last night and saw *Pretty Woman* starring Julia Roberts. I can start packing, then he'll escort me. As I stuff socks and boxers inside my rucksack, I ponder about this turn of events. I never thought being able to nip out for a paper would have seemed such a big deal.

Sprawled on his bed, Fraser is glaring. A newsagent might feel less welcoming if he was to march up to the counter. His intensity is down to his chemical imbalances, but there must be several shopkeepers who would love to relocate further up

Morningside Road, away from doped-up patients on shopping trips. I've heard the manager of the Canny Man's will bar anyone suspected of being what he would no doubt refer to as an 'escapee' caught drinking in his pub.

Ten minutes later, I watch Duncan unlock the ward door. Follow him along a labyrinthine route. I realise I haven't packed my shaving gear or toothbrush. Worrying about them seems like a Colditz escapee getting to the tunnel exit then fretting about not having made his bunk bed. We pass cleaners sharing a joke. A tuckshop queue. An attractive junior doctor whose smile makes me glow.

Ward 5 seems a world away from my previous environment: patients, including myself, haranguing staff. Screaming. Pacing the dorm at all hours. Assaulting each other. Flashing. Confusing other patients with Jesus.

Duncan leads me into the office and the charge nurse, Brigitte welcomes me, before another nurse, Claudia shows me to my dorm. She indicates the bed allocated to me. A gangly teenager sits on the next one, plugged into a Walkman. Claudia waves for him to tug out the earpieces. She introduces him. Andy.

When we shake hands, his grip is limp. But he's a psychiatric patient, not a Masonic Grand Master. He tells me his mum brought him some new cassettes last night. I can listen to some of them if I want? After I've unpacked, I reply, although that won't take long.

Claudia says she'll leave us to get acquainted. Lunch is at 12. If I feel like popping into Morningside a nurse, Maria, will chum me, at least for the first time. She'll also be running an Occupational Therapy session tomorrow.

Before she departs she suggests I phone home to let them know I've changed wards in case anyone intended visiting. There's a payphone at the ward entrance. Andy offers to show me, tossing the portable player to one side.

As I follow him, I ask him who his favourite band is. He can't say. Loads. This morning he's been listening to Erasure, U2, Bowie, Jeffrey Jackson, INXS, Bobby Marley and the Wailers. Each is announced emphatically, and he demands to know if I like Bob Marley and the Wailers, making it sound confrontational.

I tell him I do, although I wouldn't say I was a massive reggae fan. John Peel plays a fair amount. I'm always reminded of occasional forays to the reggae club in the Astoria, back when my band practised further down the hill, in the basement of the old Regent Cinema. Run by a guy from Ghana, nicknamed Papa Swi, my recollection was of being subjected to eardrum-pulverising bass, amidst a fug of weed thicker than tear gas on the Bogside.

I explain to Andy I was into punk 10 years before. For my pals and me, hearing 'Police and Thieves' on the first Clash album was our springboard into reggae. Then came 'White Man in Hammersmith Palais,' and 'Guns of Brixton.' Also Ruts D.C. He admits he doesn't like punk. Blondie are okay.

Andy's a good bit younger than me. I'm thinking his impression of punk will be less the Pistols' Spunk bootleg, more

The Exploited on *Top of the Pops* in 1981, playing breakneck heavy metal in mohicans and mail-order clothes.

We arrive at the phone. Fumbling in my pockets for change, I discover them empty. I haven't needed shrapnel for some time. Now he's talking about Peter Tosh, who was with Bob Marley until he went solo. Peter died a couple of months before. When I ask what he died of, Andy tells me burglars broke into his house, kept him and some friends hostage for hours. These robbers didn't believe him when he told them he had no money. So they shot him in the head.

He hands me 20p. *Cheers, pal.* I watch him shuffling back into the ward, sliding along the linoleum tiles in his slippers. He could generate a lot of static electricity.

I lift the receiver and phone home. Mum sounds flabbergasted to be receiving a call from me. I let her know about 'my flit,' and how I'm now in Ward 5, an *open* ward. She appreciates this is a major step and her joy is tangible, more than making up for the way my hands are trembling as I grip the phone.

I tell her about Andy, my new friend, and our musical connection. Perhaps she could bring along my Walkman on their next visit. Anne could dig out a selection of cassettes? When she asks which ones, I say to just grab a handful. A lucky dip.

*

The dorm light is extinguished, leaving the orange aura highlighting the fire exit. Andy is already heavy breathing, his manic routine of pacing the ward succumbing to fatigue.

I'm aware of a lighter's fleeting glint. Acrid smoke. Turning to my right I see a tiny glow. Luke, the pensioner in the dorm's other bed, draws from a roll-up. Moments later Claudia paces into the bedroom. She admonishes him, confiscating his Old Virginia pouch and ashtray.

I fumble for the Walkman, donning the headphones. I grasp one of the cassettes Anne handed over during the evening's visit, a dozen or so bundled inside a John Menzies carrier bag. As well as digging out a bunch of my John Peel recordings, she compiled a couple of mixtapes.

Fitting the cassette inside, my mind drifts to a book about Dachau concentration camp I once browsed through in the Napier College library – a slim but powerful volume any Holocaust denier should've been forced to read with their eyes prised open, *Clockwork Orange*-style. This covered the rise of Hitler's cult, from Brownshirts, book pyres and Kristallnacht through to obscene images of children being led away to 'showers,' mounds of emaciated corpses, and the horrible aftermath of human guinea pigs being abused in quack medical experiments.

But one photograph blew my mind. This depicted prisoners in striped overalls escorting one of their own. To the gallows. They were all playing instruments. Violins. Accordions. A clarinet. The appalling, cruel irony. The only time the inmates would have been exposed to uplifting music was when some poor soul was being led to their death. Other than that brief outburst of melody, the wretched existence of the Third Reich's brutalised victims would've been characterised by crushing silence, broken by racial slurs barked in an unfamiliar language. Guard dogs snarling. Jackboots pounding. Rifle cracks. A rope jerking. Music and silence. Life and death.

Around the same time, I wrote a philosophy essay about music. I still recall some of the quotes I used. Leo Tolstoy: "Music is the shorthand of emotion." Jane Austen: "Without music, life would be a blank to me." Jack Kerouac: "The only truth is music."

My finger jabbing 'play' brings me back, ready to quash the silence. After so long in a self-enforced, noiseless bubble of apathy, into a universe of aural sensations.

The hiss of the blank tape. John Peel's cordial voice. Muffled. But era-defining. Intrinsic to my formative teenage tastes.

I was fortunate to meet him once. Last year, I was making my way to a bus stop in Princes Street when I spotted him. Catching up, I called out: *John Peel?* About turning, he nodded. We shook hands.

There, next to Waverley Market, John Peel and I chatted. He was on his way to the station after watching New Order at the Playhouse. I gushed about how much I loved his radio show. This would be a spiel he must've heard a thousand times. But he was so self-effacing and unpretentious he just smiled, engaging with me as if I was an old friend. After we parted I realised I'd forgotten to mention Little Big Dig. If I'd had a demo on me, he would've accepted it, giving it a listen during his journey. Championing undiscovered music is in his DNA.

Fittingly, the compilation commences with The Undertones. Damian O'Neill's strident riff launches 'Listening In,' from a Peel session I recorded in January 1979, when listening into his show was a distraction from school in the morning.

The euphoric fusion of power chords and Feargal Sharkey's falsetto voice, the sound Peel adores and insists he wants played at his funeral. Set against the insane backdrop of 'The Troubles,' the Derry band provide a snapshot of joy. If the dark, the yin, is represented by Stiff Little Fingers' songs of barbed wire and Armalite rifles, The Undertones are the yang, the light, enthusing about excitement and first crushes. Teenage Kicks.

I'm transported to my teenage bedroom. Hooked on these sounds as they are being beamed live, my homework abandoned. I harness the memory. As I bask in the immaculate punk-pop, I visualise pencil marks by the door which gauged childhood bursts in height. Among the posters and ticket stubs, traces of Blue Tack are also visible in the white woodchip wallpaper, a ghostly constellation indicating where older posters hung.

In my mind, I pin these up again. Black Sabbath's *Technical Ecstasy*. Gene Simmons of Kiss, stage blood drooling from his tongue. Then, my musical tastes having undergone a seachange, clippings scissored from *Sounds* and *NME* of every band from Alternative TV to Zounds.

I think about the countless hours I escaped by listening to John Peel, how the tastes of a forty-something Merseysider were so influential on a Scottish youth. I would wait in anticipation, fingers poised on the play/record buttons of my HiFi, safe in the knowledge he never spoke over the intro or outro of any songs, allowing pristine recordings. I've dozens of tapes, reflecting the man's eclectic tastes. Punk. Post-punk. Reggae. Prog. Metal. Industrial. Acid house. Electronica. Soul. Hip-hop. Indie. Dream pop. Psychedelic pop. African pop. Iggy Pop.

Next, from a session recorded in November 1978, just over nine years ago but still sounding fresh. Crisis. 'White Youth.' The title sounds like they could be some hideous far-right band barking Aryan supremacist gibberish. But the sentiment is the polar opposite. The delivery is dynamic. Single notes and harmonics. Not bar chords. The emphatic chorus says it all: *We are black, we are white, together we are dynamite.*

Peel's voiceover: Well, I must say that of all the contemporary varieties of rock music, it's this basic and direct variety that I like the best myself.

I picture the South London punks. Shorn hair. DMs. Attitude. The aggression of Millwall supporters but instead of focused on tribal nihilism, turned against the establishment and the fascist thugs who always disrupted their gigs.

The inner sleeve of their *Hymns of Faith* mini-album portrayed the band members wearing outlaw masks. Anne took a snap of 4 Minute Warning aping this pose on the stairs at home.

This segues into a recording from two years later, September 1980. 'Shack Up,' by Manc funksters, A Certain Ratio. I've also captured a snippet of Peel murmuring about his most beloved band of all.

One thing you can say about The Fall, at least they still seem to be practising what they preached two or three years ago. There aren't many bands that can say that.

He goes on to play 'I Travel,' from *Empires and Dance*, Simple Minds' just-released third album. A mere three years on from their inception as Glasgow punks Johnny & the Self-Abusers, renamed after a Bowie lyric from 'The Jean Genie,' they've further reinvented themselves with this anthemic slice of Euro-disco.

I'm transported to Outer Limits, the early 1980s nightclub that evolved from Edinburgh's fabled punk venue, Clouds. Now a mainstream 'discotheque,' its expansive dancefloor was the perfect backdrop for this sweeping track.

Although most of my weekends were spent in the much smaller alternative venue upstairs, the Hooch, where you'd have been more likely to be assailed by the band's former incarnation's only single, 'Saints and Sinners,' along with psycho-billy outbursts, or Cabaret Voltaire's 'Nag Nag Nag,' Simple Minds merged into the stomping disco music.

We knew one of the girls who took the Hooch entry money, Giles, the gorgeous flame-haired singer from the band Hey! Elastica. She always let us in without paying, my mate Colin, Little Big Dig's first bassist, claiming this was because they were an item once. Hey! Elastica released four singles and an album. Their guitarist, Barry, went to my Sunday School when we were kids. It never ceases to amaze me how often paths cross in a capital city of half a million people.

I'd wait until later on, when the bouncers locked the doors, then sneak downstairs, and through a side entrance that connected to the Outer Limits foyer, gatecrashing 'Europe's first laser disco,' with its more expansive pool of single females.

One time I was shuffling below the trippy light show when the DJ started spinning Sister Sledge's 'We Are Family.' This exuberant soul song was adopted by the Hibs Boys as an unofficial anthem, The Family being their firm's nom-de-plume. As teenagers wrapped in Burberry and Aquascutum scarves infiltrated the dancefloor, I'd nod to faces I recognised from college.

I flip the cassette over. The following song takes me to a different continent, sunnier climes. Zimbabwe. The Bhundu Boys, 'Rugare.' Exhilarating pop, featuring their so-called jit-jive guitars, not too far removed from Johnny Marr's fluent fretwork. John Peel spoke of seeing them perform in a college in Chelsea for the first time alongside fellow Radio 1 DJ Andy Kershaw, and breaking down in tears at what he described as the most natural flowing music he had ever heard in his life. Their singer, Biggie Tembo had been a *bhundu boy*, one of the youths who assisted the guerrilla fighters opposing Ian Smith's white minority regime in Rhodesia. This summer they supported Madonna over three nights at Wembley Stadium. Some life journey. From skulking in the African bush, one eye out for army patrols, to strolling onto the stage before a combined audience of a quarter of a million spectators.

Peel championing The Bhundu Boys sent me on a journey of exploration into other bands from that continent. I went on to buy an album, prosaically entitled *African Music*. But the tunes were mesmerising, track after track of soaring guitar riffs driven by drums, bongos, brass, woodwind, xylophones, and indigenous instruments, played by flamboyant musicians named Prince Nico Mbarga, Cardinal Rex Lawson and his Majors Band of Nigeria, Dr Victor Olaiya and his International Stars Band.

The effortless melodies were made all the more poignant by the fact this was essentially Nigerian music, some songs dating to the early 1970s when many band members were lost to the Biafran War. Some of the solos I concocted for Little Big Dig were majorly influenced by The Bhundu Boys on Peel and that album.

I feel myself drifting as the next song segues. 'Venus in Furs,' from *The Velvet Underground and Nico*, the Velvets' debut, Lou Reed fantasizing about shiny boots of leather and a whiplash girl in the dark.

John Cale's violin refrain propelling the haunting track, I mime along with the Welsh maestro for a while. Grinning as I recall the serrating noise of violin lessons at Craiglockhart, under the tutelage of Mr McKinlay who smoked a pipe while listening.

My limbs feel heavy. Before sinking into sleep, I picture those same Dachau musicians playing violins. Except this time it's to celebrate the gates crashing open as American GIs liberated them all.

34

Relax

The occupational therapist, Maria invites us to sink into the beanbags. Picture our favourite food. I recall a conversation with my cousin Ross, who studied microbiology at Aberdeen University. He was a close friend of Colin Angus, guitarist in Alone Again Or. When his band swapped indie for house, re-inventing themselves as The Shamen, Colin dropped out of Uni. In a matter of months, he'd become a global pop star. But Ross explained they'd a mate up there who was obsessive about egg mayonnaise sandwiches. These would be what would tempt him back from the edge of a building in the event of any hypothetical suicide attempt rather than some negotiator's impassioned pleas.

Everyone has their equivalent of egg mayonnaise sand-wiches. Perhaps not for such drastic circumstances. For a long time, my own was a dish Mum used to throw together consist-ing of pan-fried potato slices, drenched in cheese, smothered in onions. Cheese and potato bake. I always requested this for birthday meals. Now I'm imagining having been presented with a plate, the aroma wafting, the melted cheddar still sizzling atop the charred potatoes.

Fill your minds with the thought of what it tastes like. Its delicious smell. Then think of biting into it. Think of the taste. Those wonderful flavours. Relax even more. Let your beanbag become a lilo, drifting on crystal clear waters. Any waters at all, you decide. Could be the Caribbean. Could be the Commie Pool. But wherever it is, it's just you, your floating beanbag, and the thought of the supper waiting for you.

Now Maria tells us she's going to add music. *Let this track enrich your relaxation. Try not to fall asleep. By all means feel yourselves drifting along with the lilo, the water, the soft motion of the currents, the sunshine. But try and enjoy the sensation as long as you can.*

I glance around. The others are curled into their beanbags in a variety of poses. As soon as Andy's head melted into the fabric he went out like a light. But his snores are cut out when Maria presses 'play' on her portable cassette player. 'Albatross' by Fleetwood Mac.

Listen to the relaxing sounds. Take deep, lingering breaths. The air you're breathing in, the oxygen, is pure. Draw it into the corners of your lungs. Think of your worries, your anxieties, as the carbon dioxide you're exhaling. Deep breath in. Hold it. Then release all those negative thoughts. And keep focusing on the music. This piece is called Albatross. It makes me think of a majestic bird, wings outstretched, coasting over the Southern

Ocean, a vast, grey swell, far, far below. There are churning waters down there, but up here, amongst the clouds, she's safe... she's so safe...

The plaintive guitar line breaking in makes it easy to visualise this scene. I think of its real-life equivalent. At this precise moment, as I sink deeper into this luxuriant material in a psychiatric hospital in the Scottish capital, an albatross will be gliding between remote islands never touched by human footprints, 12-foot wingspan coasting with the currents. As I drift into sleep I become that huge bird, arms outstretched, soaring through clouds.

*

After feeding my lunch tray into the clearing trolley, I head through to the dorm. Stretching back on the bed, I shut my eyes. Footsteps stomp along the corridor and there's a knock at the door. I open my eyes to see an unfamiliar guy standing over me. His badge says: Dr Philip Calvert. When he introduces himself and asks how I'm feeling, I shrug.

Okay, I mumble. Was gonna have forty winks.

He looks to the lined A4 pad Anne brought in last night, untouched on a desk.

You just do that, Mark. He swivels on his heel.

35

A Flash

This is the first time I've been entrusted to leave the ward unescorted so it's a big deal. It feels so weird stepping into the outside world after the prolonged isolation. Following Claudia's directions, each time I turn a corner I'm assailed by mundane but captivating scenes. I find myself taking in every-day activities with a sense of childlike wonder. Like E.T.

I pass posters. INXS at the Playhouse. Suzanne Vega at the Usher Hall. It feels as if I'm being readmitted to a world I'd been barred from. I pass chattering junior doctors. Whistling cleaners. Apprehensive visitors. Drugged up patients with minders, lumbering along in slippers.

Security staff steer a drunk towards the main entrance. As they usher him past, I catch a reek of his breath. Recognise him. The guy admitted to the IPCU late one night.

I find the church centre, pay 20p to the volunteer at the door. Someone else pours a mug of tea. I shovel in three sugars.

Entering the dark hall I take a seat near the back. Gaze around. The room seems vast. The soundtrack is too loud. Distorting. Indistinct. The film is set in a convent. I recognise Jane Fonda, investigating a murder. Anne Bancroft as the Mother Superior.

From an abandoned leaflet on the floor, I discover the title. *Agnes of God.* But jumping in halfway through the narrative, squinting at a screen slithering in and out of focus, I haven't a clue what's going on. I persevere for the simple reason I'm away from the ward. I could be sitting on my own in *The Dominion* further up Morningside Road. And for the feature's remaining half-hour that's where I pretend I am.

*

After I've said goodbyes to Mum, Dad, and Anne, I listen to their receding footfall. Grasp the notebook and pen Anne left. Sitting at the desk, I flip the pad open, glaring at the pristine A4 sheet with its intimidating blank lines.

Along with my musical appreciation, my urge to write anything has long been dormant. But I glance at my Walkman, the fantastical device that now transports me back to a treasure trove of memories, pointing the way forward to the light at the end of a long, bleak tunnel. Perhaps I could jot down inspirational lyrics. Even just song titles. Or a short story.

An idea formulating, I scribble a title. INK. Conjure a teenage lad. Like myself at that age, he's quiet. A bit of a loner. Somehow he's found himself in the subway beneath the railway near Saughton Park.

I've been through this tunnel myself many times, visiting my pal, Grum. Comparing records. Swapping badges.

Amongst the graffiti, I recall: THE ACCIDENTS. GRUM. ARTHUR. SHUG. BILLY. Someone painted over most of this; all that survived was GRUM ART. Like some contemporary artist from Balgreen. Suppose that's how many observers regarded punk back in 1977. Performance art of varying merit. Although the older spectators who walked out of The Accidents' anarchic debut gig in Gorgie War Memorial hall regarded this new music as the artistic equivalent of a defaced subway.

Back to my story. He clocks a much older slogan. Towards the curved ceiling. YOUNG GORGIE DERRY. 1690.

Jumping up, he scores lines through this legend with the spraypaint tin he smuggled from art class at St Augustine's that afternoon. Livid slashes. Now he writes YBT. BROOMIE BOYS. Dripping to the concrete paving. Weaving around his wrists. Green. He imagines alien blood.

Gruff voices. Someone ghosted past while he was creating his art. Figures stand either on side of him in the tunnel. He recognises them. His age. Different school. Realising his predicament, his heart pummels.

I'm picturing a wildlife documentary I once saw. Industrial fishing in the Barents Sea. A massive trawler winched up vast lines, hundreds of hooks glinting in the murky depths. Every barb impaling a tiny squid. As these creatures were hauled from their habitat, up to the horrible dancing lights, each one puffed out ink. Millennia of evolution controlling their instinctive defence mechanisms. Deterring danger. Hundreds of tiny bursts of black ink. Impotent. Pointless. Every brief cloud a lifeform being killed.

Like one of the squids, the lad digs his trembling finger into the nozzle. A hiss. Flashing against the striplights, a blade. He feels a fist dig into his side. Searing pain. The cold, grey pathway rushing up. Taking his breath away.

Hello, Mark. How are you doing?

Startled, I drop the pen. Turn to see my latest visitor. Keith Robinson. I check his white moustache and his dog collar.

Fine... Mr Robinson. I didn't expect to see you.

He tugs out a spare chair. Your mum's been keeping me up to speed, Mark. I was sorry to hear you've not been well. But you're looking fit and healthy.

A little fazed, I nod. I'm much better, thanks.

As a child, Sunday School was something Anne and I *had* to go to, like Monday to Friday school. After the morning class, you filed into the main hall for a portion of the service, returning before the main session.

When you got older and had to sit right through, you'd watch the Minister plodding up the steps to the top pulpit and launch into a protracted lesson. Firebrand preachers might have been able to arrest the attention of the most sceptical onlookers. Mr Robinson's sermons were delivered in an affable but soporific monotone. I suspected few of his congregation managed to follow the obscure, twisting paths of his existential preaching to arrive at the conclusion. The message.

I stopped going to church when my life began revolving around punk gigs and the Saturday binges necessitating Sunday lie-ins.

Mum still goes. Recently she became a deacon. But returning from evening meetings she moans about the petty politics. Personality clashes. North Merchiston Church's finances are in disarray. Elders consistently bicker. One sneers at her when she speaks. Cut from the same cloth as John Knox, the medieval misogynist whose literal interpretation of God's word bemoaned women having any position of authority.

We spend 15 or so minutes chatting. Mostly me listening, but so what? Mum once told me his wife had some mental health condition that remained undiagnosed. I'm grateful he was thinking of me.

Standing, he gives a firm handshake. Says he'll drop by again. Soon.

I get a hint of cigarettes on his breath and notice the yellowy tinge to his moustache. I suspect he's eager to light up as soon as he reaches his car. He might wear a white collar but he's only human.

Keith Robinson has been a family friend for years. I can even recall the day he dipped his finger into the font and traced a cross over my forehead, then Anne's. For some reason, our christening was delayed and we were toddlers rather than babies.

Religion may have long evaporated from my life to be replaced by a less dogmatic, humanist sense of spiritualism. But his unexpected visit is nothing but a friendly reassurance.

*

My eyes adjusting to the gloom, I fish into the bag, grasp a cassette. It's a mixtape, Anne's choice. Stifling the harsh stereo of Luke and Andy's snores, I press 'play'. This erupts into the crunching goose-step intro to 'Holidays in the Sun.' The Sex Pistols. A pivotal song.

Paul Cook's drumming. Glen Matlock's melodic basslines. Steve Jones' majestic Gibson Les Paul power chords and intricate licks. Johnny Rotten's caustic vocal delivery. Rotten, the most obvious face of the punk scene, pouring scorn on a world where, out of all the British Isles' working-class patronised and discriminated against, Irish immigrants would always be denigrated most of all. Forced to endure everything from Irish jokes to 'No Irish, No Blacks, No Dogs,' notices pinned to post-war London guesthouses.

The band inspired tabloid hysteria. Furious letters to the *Daily Mail.* Censorship from airplay. Dumping by two major record labels. I recall one of the countless snooty reviews dismissing *Never Mind the Bollocks, Here's The Sex Pistols* as 'cockney war chants.' The multicultural unity of their fans was sometimes a focal point for lumpen National Front violence.

But they were merely following a chain of quintessentially English rock 'n' roll dating back to The Kinks and Small Faces. Cattle-prodded by The New York Dolls, The Stooges, and The Ramones from over the pond.

Next, The Damned. 'Sick Of Being Sick.' Apt. I bought their debut album *Damned Damned Damned* after school from Hot Wax in Dalry Road, when there were record shops all over the city. It encapsulated punk's raucousness but listening to Brian James' frenetic soloing made you appreciate his skills. Like Steve Jones. Mick Jones. Hugh Cornwell. Paul Weller. Stuart Adamson. John McGeoch. Punk bands might have stripped everything right back, transforming the energy of the rock bands that had preceded them into three-minute outbursts, but nothing was dumbed down in the process. These guys could play.

Next, grassroots punk, the simple two-note riff introducing 'I'm An Upstart,' by Angelic Upstarts. Transports me to their gig at Heriot-Watt Student Union in Grindlay Street, May 1979. Supported by Metropak, who practised in Blair Street alongside The Axidents.

Having chosen to leave school, I hadn't achieved good enough Higher passes for the Edinburgh University history degree I'd applied for. But had no idea about the alternatives. I chose to switch off from fretting about an uncertain future and pogo the night away like a demented jack-in-the-box.

At one point their stage crew produced a severed pig's head from a carrier bag, an unsubtle manifestation of their anti-police stance. This macabre bruised and bloody lump was tossed around the crowd, striking my mate, Grum as he was lighting a fag.

Now Suzanne Vega. New York folk-rock. I'd never listened to her until Andy loaned me his cassette of *Solitude Standing*. Now Anne has bought the album for me and taped one of the tracks, 'Calypso.' Halfway in, a spiralling guitar solo raises my spirits so much I rewind. And again.

I'm already drifting towards sleep when the cassette clicks to a halt. I tug the earphones away and they clatter to the floor, just in time to hear the mischievous pensioner rummaging in his bedside drawer before lighting another rollup. Johnny Rotten would've approved.

36

Hash City Rockers and Red Hands

December 1987

Mid-day sunlight streams through the windows. Seated before me are a group of students, all several years my junior. At their centre, an affable older woman regards me through red-rimmed glasses and offers the vacant chair. The psychiatrist introduces herself as Dr Atkinson and commences by thanking me for agreeing to this session. She underlines this is just an informal chat to give her students a taste of conducting an assessment. Receiving an insider's view would be invaluable to their training.

Referring to my case notes, she observes it has only been a few weeks since my admission to the IPCU suffering from an acute psychotic episode. Glancing at the ironed 501s and petrol blue Next shirt Mum handed over during last night's visit, she mentions my recovery seems to be progressing well. She draws my attention to the video camera perched on a tripod in the background, its recording light blinking red.

She throws questions to the floor. A female at the back raises her hand. Enquires if recreational drugs were an influence? I admit to a fondness for the amber nectar. This produces a ripple of empathy. Medical students are alleged to binge like AC/DC roadies. A male colleague enquires whether I smoked a lot of cannabis.

My intake would be best described as modest. Intermittent. Scorned by many I know. I remember Ronnie Dudgeon, a stout, jocular guy from Stenhouse from the punk days, whom I'd bump into crossing Harrison Park en route to Napier while he was striding to a building site in Polwarth. He was always toking on the fat spliff he described as *breakfast*, his hilarious stories lapsing into protracted coughing fits. One sticking in my mind was the time he'd taken so much speed at a party, instead of dancing to The Pogues with everyone else, he set off for a jog around Carrick Knowe golf course at half three in the morning, *like a fucking fat Bionic Man. Hydroponic Man!* Like many in Edinburgh, he didn't make it past the 1980s after progressing to heroin and sharing needles.

Rather than casting up Ronnie as a comparison, I admit to occasional weekend joints between pubs. More often when I was playing in bands.

I remember 4 Minute Warning practices in the dingy cellars beneath the derelict Regent Cinema. We were just kids. All still living at home. But this was our den.

Peering around, I wonder about mentioning my punk teens. I'd be broaching a subculture none of them will have much of a clue about, their perception of *punk* restricted to youths in birds-of-paradise hairstyles posing for London tourists five years after the Pistols split.

The Regent and Abbeyhill would be even further from any of their radars. And if I used the nearest pub as a compass reference – Cairns Bar, under the railway bridge, owned by Pat Stanton and Alan Gordon – I would further test my audience's attention span.

I think of the stories I could tell about getting wrecked at rehearsals. Or the time we investigated a break-in at the cinema upstairs, entering via an ancient door that had been jemmied open, discovering ticket kiosks with *£sd* prices, sloshing through puddles from roof leaks, hearing the vandals escaping into the main hall, giving chase in the stygian gloom, tumbling over broken floorboards.

Mum used to go to the Regent, one of many popular picture houses on the east side. The queues snaked down the stairs to the lower road. Sometimes air raid sirens sounded during the shows. A stray bomb struck a house in Loaning Road, round the corner from her home. Mum knew one of the sisters who died, Betty Veitch, a couple of years above her at Craigentinny secondary.

My mind is wandering way off-topic. At least I'm aware of this. Someone asked about cannabis. Hash City Rockers. Whether it's the relaxed atmosphere, the camera's remorseless scrutiny, or being invited to chat about subjects that interest me after months of being trapped inside a depressive fog, I feel inspired to unwind. To engage in conversation.

I explain the Regent shut around 1970. By 1980 it was used for rehearsal rooms. We were allocated a space alongside mates in another punk band, Sceptix, in a partitioned corridor beside the cinema's former boiler room, now a communal dumping ground and toilet.

There were no lights in that stinking anteroom, piled high with rotting fag packets, used johnnies, chippy wrappers, beer cans, bottles. Every so often you'd step to the edge of the pit to piss, adding to the raw sewage accumulating in this poisonous latter-day Nor Loch for years, from guys emulating Pink Floyd to us with our Killing Joke badges.

This cesspit always reminded me of the rubbish tip on the Death Star in *Star Wars*. Perched in the gloom, you could imagine some creature lurking. After a smoke, you'd almost *hear* tentacles slithering towards your ankles.

After our jamming sessions, we got stuck into the blow. Taking the shortcut. Beer can. Hole gouged in the top with a key. Tinfoil over it. Hash crumbs onto this. Apply a lighter. Sook from the can opening. You needed cast iron lungs.

The weird thing was, although this got you ripped, I didn't feel that way the first time. I recall heading up to the chippy on Montrose Terrace. When I came back to the room, our drummer Shug had stuck on a cassette of Gang of Four's *Entertainment* at top volume. Andy Gill's guitar was shredding my skull while I tore into a fish supper. My second in the space of half an hour.

I do still struggle to differentiate between thinking and thinking aloud. Do I want to be so candid about recreational drugs? Illegal drugs. I note the camera lens again. Feel a note of panic. Patient confidentiality? At least the memories are coherent. A snapshot of my youth. But I decide to minimise any confessional aspect.

For all that I still visualise the Regent as a murky cavern, we spent five nights out of seven practising there. The post-punk scene was still in its infancy and we relished the possibilities awaiting us each time we plugged in our equipment, with or without chemical stimulants. I also loved dreaming up lyrics. Still have some of the originals written in BT notebooks Dad gave me from his work. I added Anarchy and Peace symbols in the margin.

A guy who drank in the Regent Buffet where we retired most nights. Tam Doig. Doigy. I see him marching into the pub, tugging on a doob, a baseball bat ill-concealed behind his back, swaying over to our table and demanding to know if any of us had seen someone he referred to as Chubby. We shook our heads, willing him to move on.

In among the crap tattoos proliferating over his arms, I spotted a crimson constellation of track marks. That evening we were jamming a cover of Johnny Thunder and The Heartbreakers' 'One Track Mind.' The irony was just as overwhelming as Doigy using the innocuous nickname of someone he intended to bludgeon.

Dr Atkinson has moved on from the substances I dabbled in seven years ago. She is discussing other complex issues that impact mental health. Drugs will reduce dopamine, an organic chemical, causing an imbalance. But other factors can be a trigger. Hormone imbalances. Traumatic events, like child abuse, can prompt post-traumatic stress disorder.

Purse my lips at that. She asks if I'm going to do anything differently when discharged. Many patients take the opportunity to press the reset button. I mumble something about the Northern Ireland flag pinned to my bedroom wall.

Cause my dad's from there. Well, he's not. He's from Monaghan. The Irish Republic. Loyalists conflate the six counties with the centuries-old province, 40% of which lies over the border. You only ever see Ulster flags at Old Firm matches in the Celtic end. Would that flag have ended up there if my mind was balanced?

Blank looks. But I continue, nerves prising the words like a fissure in a dam.

Sometimes, when I was *blind* drunk, staggering home from Lothian Road in a slalom, I sang snippets of those *horrible* songs, too. The ones lurking beyond the euphemism *party pieces*. 'Rule Britannia.' 'The Sash.'

Pals and workmates, would ask: *Why? What are you coming out with that knuckle-dragging Hun crap for? That's not you. You've got Highers. Been to college. Thought you were a Shandon Hibee? A Gorgie green?*

To paraphrase the Dead Kennedys. Things happen when you're too drunk to give a fuck. Although no one gets the reference, they all laugh.

My band Little Big Dig shared a practice room with Family Von Trapp, Muriel Gray's band. They were Glasgow Art

College graduates. They'd say: *How can someone from Edinburgh, who plays these beautiful pop songs, be into that medieval nonsense?*

A girlfriend asked about that flag. She didn't recognise it. Northern Ireland, I explained. Later, she told me she described it to her flatmate who reckoned I must be in the Orange Lodge. Which meant having an issue with Catholics. She reminded me she went to Augys. St Augustine's. Asked if I hated *her*, or her family? I was *horrified* at that.

I only ever saw the flag as being a celebration of my dad's Ulster unionism, the latter very much a small 'u.' Never anti-Catholicism. Certainly never anti-Irishness. Unlike many from that side of the Irish Sea who espowsed Unionism with a stridently large 'U,' Dad was always proud to be Irish.

Splodge would just laugh at the mad incongruity of someone normally regarded as one of the good cunts having these weird lapses. But Tom hit the nail on the head. He noticed the party songs would rise in inverse proportion to my success with girls. If I left the Hooch, some gig at the Wee Red Bar, or one of the parties we gatecrashed after picking up the address in The Tap, with a girl, I'd be Jekyll. Going home alone, my failures ranging from knockbacks to an occasional slap, Hyde would stagger off into the night, his ludicrous demons mustered, crooning about Derry's Walls, if only for the few hours until Sunday's hangover.

My head is reeling. This morning's medication. What percentage of that spiel remained internal? How much slipped out?

Dr Atkinson confirms I shared a portion of my inner rambling. Removing a flag is a first, Mark! People say things like... taking up yoga. Joining a gym. This must be a subject you've been giving serious thought to. A couple of weeks ago you wouldn't have been capable of such objectivity.

A couple of weeks ago I thought the visitor room in my last ward had sprung a leak, like a spaceship, and the air was escaping.

Everyone chuckles at the absurdity. Although they're trainees, guaranteed they'll already have enough material for *volumes* of the bizarre stories divulged during these grillings.

*

Dr Calvert lifts the pad. So you're a writer, Mark?

I was, yes. Had some stories published in my local newspaper. Gorgie Gazette.

Excellent. I see you've been writing something new? That's really good, Mark. Not feeling so confused these days?

Erm, no. Just had a wee idea, about football. Airdrie away to Meadowbank, a couple of months ago. Thought I'd go with it.

Dr Calvert skims the flash short story, although I see him squinting. I had to really focus on getting my fingers to stop shaking.

Excellent, Mark. Keep this up. It's really good for your recovery, to get back into something as creative as story writing. I have a meeting with Jenny Atkinson later. I'd like to discuss getting you a weekend pass organised.

I tell him that sounds great, then he smiles and exits. Reading over the story again, scribbling adjustments, I decide I'll hand this to Anne next visiting time. She can type it for me during her lunch break.

PUNKETTE AT HAYMARKET

The next train was rammed with baying football supporters. Bedecked in red and white, the windows steamed up by their chanting were draped with Northern Ireland flags and Union Jacks, the largest version of the latter embossed with AIRDRIE LOYALISTS: posters advertising tribalism as enduring and neverending as train timetables. Appalled by their obscene gestures and Simian mating calls, she felt an an incongruous superiority, looking in on them as if they were a zoo exhibit.

One fan, his stomach a white tyre between jeans and T-shirt, hoisted himself up to reach for the window like a survivor groping for the last air pocket. As a beer can spat in punctuation in the background, his parting comments were drowned by the train's gathering momentum. He looked to be mouthing 'Embra slut!' Noticing a bespectacled boy around her son's age sitting next to him, dressed in a little replica of his team's red-V logo, she stuck her tongue out, chuckling when he returned the gesture.

*

Gazing at the night light above the door, I slide the volume up. 'Blue Monday.' New Order. Ian Curtis, Bernard Sumner and Peter Hook were inspired by The Sex Pistols' two appearances at Manchester's Free Trade Hall in the summer of 1976, a catalytic event that heralded Buzzcocks, The Fall, Magazine, Slaughter and the Dogs, and their own band, Warsaw, later Joy Division.

I took Anne to watch Buzzcocks at the Odeon in October 1979 when she was 14, with Joy Division supporting. They were still playing pre-*Unknown Pleasures* material like 'Leaders of Men,' and 'Digital.' The highlight of their raw but captivating set was Curtis's mesmeric performance, culminating in him being helped off stage.

But when the remaining members became New Order after Curtis's premature death at 23, they gatecrashed a whole new sonic dimension, taking their influences from Kraftwerk and Hi-NRG.

With its unmistakable intro, courtesy of the Oberheim DMX drum machine they'd just bought, and using a hook that Hooky admitted ripping off from a Donna Summer B-side, it became the biggest-selling 12" of all time. Described as a crucial crossover between 1970s disco and 1980s house, listening to this glorious seven-minute epic does take me back to Solution in Blair Street, a 'traditional disco' housed in the South Bridge's basement warrens, where punters from South Edinburgh's schemes often curtailed the music by engaging in furious melees on the dancefloor. Also the Hooch, one of the capital's first clubs to feature house music.

This gives way to Cocteau Twins. 'Sugar Hiccup.' Robin Guthrie's layered guitar and Elizabeth Fraser's lilting soprano conjure shimmering soundscapes. As the track nears its conclusion I'm tempted to rewind but I want to satiate my senses with the next tune.

'Genius of Love.' Tom Tom Club, a side project of Tina Weymouth, founder member and bassist of Talking Heads.

From the viewpoint of someone in a prison cell, the narrator describes her love for her sweetheart to her inmates, while paying tribute to a roll-call of genius African American performers: George Clinton, Bootsy Collins, Smokey Robinson, Hamilton Bohanon, James Brown, Bob Marley, Sly and Robbie, and Kurtis Blow. I've danced to most of the namechecked artists at the Hooch.

Following on from this, another song reminiscent of that nightclub, and one of the most sublime Scottish pop singles ever: 'Party Fears Two' by The Associates. My senses soar for the four breathtaking minutes of Billy Mackenzie's swirling voice and Alan Rankine's exultant keyboard refrain. The bittersweet tension of its beautiful melodies and Billy's lyrics about the alcohol loving you but turning you blue.

I change cassettes again. After the brash impudence of punk expanding into the infinite possibilities of post-punk, I'm turning back time.

Queen. When I was in 2nd Year, 'Bohemian Rhapsody' lodged at number one for nine weeks over the end of 1975. On Christmas Eve, BBC2 broadcast their festive gig at the Hammersmith Odeon. Together with the single, these events marked my transition from being a kid into Glam and pop to a teenage rock fan.

'Seven Seas of Rhye' was the first single I bought. Dad drove me up to Sound Centre in Clerk Street, and the 50p it cost me in 1975 seemed a big deal.

But the track blasting from the earphones is 'Brighton Rock,' the opener to their third album, *Sheer Heart Attack*. After Freddie Mercury's stunning vocals swirl through the first two verses, it launches into an exhilarating Brian May guitar solo.

A couple of years later, Queen sounded overblown, denigrated by the punk thought police as a sonic indulgence compared to the frenzied adrenaline rush of the emerging rock 'n' roll scene.

But as punk became a distant memory, much of the vinyl shoved to the back of my record collection during my teens was reinstated, Queen's early albums being granted pride of place behind Punishment of Luxury's *Laughing Academy*. The swirling escapism of his unaccompanied fretwork is perfect for how I'm feeling.

37

Psychos

I was checking the times for Glasgow Central when I saw this nutcase out the corner of my eye. He walked up to a guy, a guy in a suit, slashed his face with a small blade... like a penknife. The police caught him on Waverley Bridge. He was just released from that loony bin in Morningside. Someone should start a petition to put an electrified fence around that place. Used to be a lunatic asylum. Don't know why they changed that. I sometimes go to the Dominion. You spot the crazies with their helpers. I always move seats.

I shoot a glance at the TV. The middle-aged woman being interviewed, with a Princess Anne bouffant and a Burberry shawl, is a cliché herself.

Bryan is far more forthright. Just *listen* to her fucking crap, Mark? What a fucking *ignorant* human being.

Bryan, a nurse, is a cheery, potty-mouthed Mancunian, his life's mission championing underdogs. Like a Glaswegian favouring the Jags, the Bully Wee, or the Spiders over the Old Firm, he has eschewed his home city's red and sky blue divide, opting for Stockport County's royal blue and white.

We also have regular chats about our favourite Manc bands, from Buzzcocks, Joy Division, Magazine, and The Fall to more recent stuff, The Smiths, The Chameleons. Yesterday he unbuttoned his grey shirt to reveal a T-shirt bearing the one-time controversial sleeve image for 'Orgasm Addict,' a topless model desexualized by having her head replaced by a domestic iron. I demanded the mail order address.

Bryan's main bone of contention is his jokes tend to be wasted on his usual audience. Not through ignorance. Anti-psychotic medication isn't ideal for rapier ripostes.

He concludes by surmising her attitude to the Christmas Day truce in 1914 would've been marking the German half over a minefield.

So much for the season of fucking goodwill, Mark.

In the studio, Sheena McDonald summarises the afternoon's incident, painting a more balanced picture than the interviewee.

Bryan bemoans the blurred line between mental illness and criminality. These random attacks make headlines *because* they are exceptional. Compared to the bloodbath of GBH and attempted murder occurring every week across the country after the final whistle on Saturday afternoons, or closing time on Sunday mornings.

He reels off pseudonyms for his charges; another patient, Bill and I chip in. *Nutcases. Psychos. Bams. Nutters. Maddos.*

Crazies. Numpties. Space cadets. Loonies. Schizos. Idiots. Retards. Freaks. Spastics.

Bryan says cancer patients are cancer patients. But mental patients seem to have more synonyms than Innuits use for snow.

As he cello tapes a fairy to the treetop, he concludes Lady Burberry will have similar feelings about immigrants. Gays. The homeless. All the sensibilities of a fucking Dalek. Her attitude is fucking *worse* than the red devil or NF-tattooed skinheads he received more than the occasional beating from. She wouldn't be administering any kickings, but she seemed articulate enough to appreciate words could dish out metaphoric violence. That sticks and stones quote? Words will never hurt? Fucking nonsense.

*

It's only a visit to Morningside Library, a few minutes from the ward, but it's so much more. This is a massive deal. Strolling towards the main road, my limbs are stiff: a combination of unfamiliarity with exercise and chlorpromazine.

But as I watch a packed maroon bus trundling by, I smile. This is my first unescorted foray into the world outside the psychiatric hospital. I appreciate the symbolism. I'm several steps closer to the end of the tunnel. To wellbeing. As the looming black clouds open, I step up my pace for the final block.

Inside the library, I gaze at the cupola I recall from childhood visits. I would head straight for the dinosaur books and remember borrowing one volume and copying the text into a jotter, word for word, Latin taxonomy and all, chapter after chapter. Adding my own illustrations. I gave up by the advent of the Jurassic period.

Another infatuation was military uniforms. I would painstakingly reproduce Napoleonic soldiers in a different jotter. From British infantry and French cavalry red to Dutch, French, and Prussian blue. With all the artillery smoke wafting across the battlefields, the aiming of muskets must have become a lottery. I once sketched an officer of the Brunswick Corps, German troops who dressed in black with skull and crossbones insignia, like some proto-SS unit. Except they fought in Wellington's army.

I was equally obsessed with redcoats on the big screen. Mum would take me to see *Zulu*, *The Charge of the Light Brigade*, and *Waterloo*, at the Tivoli in Gorgie, or The Dominion, where I'd be amongst the youngest audience members. After watching *Waterloo*, I drew the doomed charge of the Scots Greys in crayons. This remains in a frame amongst the gallery in the front room at home, next to the oldest surviving example of my artwork, a yellow submarine inspired by The Beatles' song I loved listening to on the radio. I would have been about four.

When I was studying at Napier, searching for books to complement the English Literature coursework, I would drift towards Scottish fiction. I recall standing in this very spot and reading a short by James Kelman, 'Forgetting to Mention Allende.'

Roving over the rich array of titles, I spot *The Big Man*, by William McIlvanney. Easing it from the shelf, I skim the blurb.

It's about a miner and prizefighter, a reviewer waxing lyrical about the bare-knuckle prose. I take it to the counter.

The cloudburst is petering out by the time I reach the hospital entrance, the paperback clutched inside my jacket. Before I turn the corner, a white van speeds by. I catch two guys slouched behind the grubby windscreen, *The Sun* poked into the dashboard.

Spot the looney... spot, spot, spot, spot the loooooney! reverberates from the passenger-side window.

*

Bryan places the scissors down and brushes the excess hair from my shoulders. Crouches to peer into the mirror level with my haircut. He asks whether I like my haircut, or am I going to sue him?

Glaring into the reflection, I make it seem like I'm considering this, then grin. I'm beaming, and tell him he could get a job at Brian Drumm's if he gets fed up with psychiatric nursing. Nodding, he explains he was a hairdresser for five years in Bury before deciding to switch from dealing with the outside of the head to the inside.

Claudia appears, informs me my sister has arrived to do some Christmas shopping. Detouring to my bedroom, I grab a jacket. Anne grins when I bound into the meeting room, admiring the new look, reminding me Mum used to refer to my wilder locks as 'The Wild Man of Borneo.' I comment I heard somewhere there *was* a Wild Man of Borneo, some wrestler from the 1960s. Probably came from no further east than Tranent.

Ten minutes later, we're dipping in and out of the shops on Morningside Road, against a backdrop of Slade, Wizzard, Wham, Band Aid. Rather than wrapping a few main gifts for our folks, we always cram a bunch of items into stockings. Dad's face lights up when he delves deep to recover the first presents packed: Carlsberg Special tins.

Anne pats my shoulder, wonders what I would've been doing this time last year?

I tell her I had a ticket for the party in Buster Brown's. We got a half day from work. I spent all afternoon in the Traveller's Tryst. Got a number 4 home to change and shower. Fell asleep. Woke at the Fairmilehead terminus. Then I got the bus straight back into town. Madogs. Busters. Unconscious in a corner and ejected by the bouncers by half eleven.

Doesn't sound like much fun, Mark, she says. Hardly the season to be jolly.

This season's going to be better. Defo.

*

Brigit, the Charge Nurse, is the antithesis of those starchy, spinster-like, navy-blue uniformed sisters that prowled the wards in *Carry On* films. Rosy-cheeked and plump, she speaks with a rich Dublin brogue that lapses into chuckles. If she has to be assertive, she drops that affable accent an octave. You could imagine this mellow Blarney taking seconds to have a snarling Rottweiler imploring to have its tummy tickled. She indicates the spare seat opposite her desk.

She pauses while she considers my opened file. It seems an incongruous tome for someone still young enough for Club

18-30 holidays. But she informs me Dr Calvert, the house registrar, is so pleased with my progress that he's recommended a weekend pass. I can spend Christmas at home.

Brigit pauses, smiling as my face lights up like a Christmas tree. She tells me I return on the twenty-eighth for a couple of days. Then, if all goes well, I can go home for the New Year. For good.

When I blurt out my joy at my imminent release, she guffaws and lets me know the customary expression is *discharged*. Not only was this an open ward, the time has long gone when psychiatric hospitals were maximum-security prisons with fewer syllables.

But I'm pragmatic enough to realise a discharge marks the end of phase one of treatment. The most intense phase. The transition has to be handled with care. I have aspirations to reclaim my place as a functional member of society. But it's only been days since I was doped up to the eyeballs with a cocktail of psychiatric mood suppressants. So my period as an outpatient will begin with Christmas with my family, as good a place to start picking up the pieces as any.

When I go home, I'll start self-medicating. She insists I'll have to be conscientious about taking my tablets when not on the ward. Nobody wants me to relapse. I nod. A small price to pay for being given permission to walk out the hospital's front door and back into my life.

38

Pills 'N' Thrills And Straightjackets

May 1988

In the hospital, patients referred to chlorpromazine as 'the chemical straightjacket.' When I was first given this drug in the IPCU my doses were administered as an oral syrup, the orange spoonfuls reminding me of custard, a childhood favourite. I became curious. Looked it up in a medical dictionary in my local library, Fountainbridge.

"*Chlorpromazine. The world's first antipsychotic, introduced in 1950. From a family of neuroleptics, principally used to treat schizophrenia, bipolar disorder, and attention deficit hyperactivity disorder, it also calms patients before surgery. Each member of this chemical family has subtly different effects on consciousness but chlorpromazine counters many of the symptoms of psychotic illness, especially phantom voices, paranoid delusions, and hallucinations.*

Like any drug, medicinal or recreational, it has powerful side effects. Impaired vision. Respiratory problems. Lethargy. Long-term usage can lead to liver damage. Chlorpromazine patients are often characterised by a zombie-like demeanour; the drug has earned its nom-de-plume because of one particular side-effect: reversible but deeply unpleasant muscle-stiffening."

Having taken my ration of chlorpromazine tablets an hour before, I sense the straightjacket constricting my body after each mouthful of rum and ginger. This glutinous solution does provide a medicinal but sugar-coated hit, putting me in mind of something that might have been administered to psychiatric patients during those notorious CIA experiments in the 1950s. But it also leaves a pleasant honeyed aftertaste.

I'm *compos mentis* enough to be pondering the advisability of blending so much alcohol with the meds in my bloodstream but Big Country are thundering from the HiFi speakers, and after clocking my depleted glass Alex is mixing our next round of doubles in-between air guitaring to Stuart Adamson and Bruce Watson's duelling fretwork.

The room is rocking, enough to drive away the lingering sense of paranoia I still face when contemplating hitting rammed nightspots a mere five months after incarceration in a psychiatric unit.

I slug at my Red Stripe, alternating with Alex's current chaser of choice: OVD Demerara Rum and Crabbie's Green

Ginger Wine. Rocket fuels as he describes this brain cell oblit-erating concoction. I appreciate the medical staff who were so meticulous in writing out my case notes might not appreciate my rehabilitation being treated in such a cavalier fashion. In the history of remedies, no medication has ever been prescribed without a proviso about avoiding alcohol.

But that swaying sensation, the raucous post-punk back-drop, and the thought of horned-up gangs of single women prowling Lothian Road is an intoxicating fusion. That dous-ing the chlorpromazine tablets I swallowed just before Alex arrived is akin to pouring gasoline onto a fire ceased being a warning long ago. Now it's more like Russian roulette, only with a slim possibility of casual sex to accompany the head wasting blows of the lager and rum chasers.

Putting out a fire, with gasoline. Bowie's song comes to me, from the film *Cat People*. Malcolm McDowell. Natassja Kinski. Directed by Roman Polanski. Alex was discussing him earlier. Polanski was rattling Kinski when she was 15. Before that, he was charged with the statutory rape of a 13-year-old girl he was photographing in Jack Nicholson's house after plying her with quaaludes.

Film directors or Rolling Stones bassists can get away with abusing minors. Anyone else would be added to a sex register. Alex concluded that after what happened to Sharon Tate and their unborn child, his moral compass must've taken a jolt.

When I stand up to accept the three arrows Alex has just plucked from the dartboard, the floor heaves like a ship's deck. Although we're still hours from any nightclub, my head is already spinning. This was the routine in the months before my illness, and resuming where I left off seems the most appropriate reaction to what was a temporary hiatus. Much as any medical professional will underline alcohol is a potent anti-depressive, they surely place some credence in an ex-patient wishing to return to 'normal'? This is what I keep trying to convince myself.

I'm going for treble 18. That I'm seeing two versions of this red segment renders the task hopeless. Alex cracks something about my first throw being about as close to their intended target as the Belgrano was to the Royal Navy exclusion zone during the Falklands War. My second misses the board, puncturing a *Sounds* cutting of Mark E Smith, right in his plums. I sing a helium-voiced version of 'Industrial Estate.'

The way we both cackle is far more demented than it deserves, but I'm viewing this Friday night in the context of recapturing my pre-breakdown lifestyle. Recovery over relapsing. So many 'normal' young adults in any Scottish town or city use their weekends for getting hammered.

Chaotic darts and loud guitars were always the backdrop to draining Victoria Wine carryouts, charging ourselves before the shock of the city centre bar prices. Tonight we've been knocking back Red Stripes – a rare ostentatious choice given these were the first lagers to break the £1 barrier a couple of years back – and are swigged straight from the can in uptown bars as if aspirational trendies feel the need to remind themselves of underage sessions on park benches.

The dark rum and ginger nips offer a cloyingly sweet taste, conjuring the thrill of pre-Merky youth club booze ups when you fortified yourself for an evening of pogoing to The Damned's 'Neat Neat Neat,' 999's 'I'm Alive,' and Wire's '12XU,' while staring at the streetlights moshing over the Union Canal's ripples.

The initial slurps gave a satisfying glow. By the fourth serving, our smiles were becoming rigid as clowns. By our eighth, we were roaring intense nonsense and missing doubles around the board. We would've struggled to hit two sperm whales beached at Portobello.

When we take our drinking session uptown our first port of call is the ABC cinema's upstairs lounge bar. As well as offering promotional shorts at prices from around the time *The Exorcist* was terrifying audiences, this watering hole is situated at the vortex of Lothian Road, Morrison Street, and Bread Street. From here pub crawls can head northwards towards Rose Street's 'amber mile' of 12 bars, westwards to the Tollcross nightclubs, or eastwards to the West Port's three Go-Go bars – Edinburgh's 'pubic triangle.'

After four more rounds, we fire over the road to Morrison's, around the corner to Lothian Road, onto Lord Tom's then Palmer's, and last of all, The Amphitheatre. Smaller than its Roman namesake, gladiators often engage in combat or seek virgins for sacrifice with equal gusto. Except for me.

After the supreme effort of standing parade ground straight to give the door staff a false impression of sobriety, I'm ensconced in a corner of the dancehall. Gawking at the disco lights sparkling against an untouched pint of lager losing its fizz before my bleary eyes. Concentrating on the rhythmic breathing I'm convinced will pre-empt regurgitation of my stomach contents. Any time a prowling bouncer hoves into view, Alex seizes the scruff of my neck to hold me upright, like I'm his ventriloquist dummy.

'What You Need' by INXS blares over the sound system. Alex tells me this is my song because I'm so *in excess* that lager is starting to fucking leak from my ears.

As I almost manage to snort at this vision, he clambers to his feet, announcing it's high time I gave myself a shake before pestering 'a couple of tidies.' My defence that I'm cunted and need to ride it out for a bit is ignored. As he hauls me up, further protest is impossible. My tongue has become lodged to the roof of my mouth with a glue tasting of honey.

He marshals me into the dense throng, selecting a pair of females and positioning me before one. While Michael Hutchence croons something masquerading as a romantic song but which is all about the bulge in his leather trousers, I attempt to wiggle my hips to the Australian rockers.

I scan other blokes on the dancefloor, although my vision reveals far more than there are, and the motion hurts my eyes. I'm reminded of the motley collection of males in David Attenborough films, where everything from Fijian parrots to Galapagos iguanas are obligated to pass an audition process: seconds of bizarre body language that will decide whether or not there will be any sex in due course.

I check out Alex. The moment he tapped his partner's bare shoulder and she responded with a coy smile, he seized the opportunity. Now he's stopped dancing, leaning in to bellow into his victim's ear. She grins at his inane sweet nothings.

My partner has a perplexed expression. Perhaps she's wondering why I'm not spoon-feeding her my own chat-up lines. Worse than that, she might've got the impression I only tagged along to make up numbers. Nothing could be further from the truth. She's an attractive woman, early twenties. Beautiful eyes twinkling beneath a sleek black bob. Her emphatic make-up reminds me of Siouxsie Sioux circa 'Love in a Void.' Without the swastikas.

Alex catches my eye. Fires a poisonous look. Because the truth of the situation is this. No matter how much of an impression he is making, even if she's smitten with his charm, her prime loyalty will be to her friend. And if her friend hasn't clicked in the same way, then the moment this record merges into the next they'll move on to the next two likely lads. Few girls get so besotted with drunken chat they'd abandon a mate. Guys do that all the time, accept this as part of the ritual. But if I fail this audition, so does Alex.

Growing more agitated, he breaks off from the dance. Grasps my collar. Insists I chat up 'the pal,' as 'his yin' is eating out his hand. He says this loud enough for his dancing partner to hear how she is eating out of his hand.

The music gets louder. The beat pounds my senses. The overhead lights flare as if I've stumbled too close to a firework display.

A hangover from my teenage days is an incessant need to analyse music, dismissing bands or artists I regard as lacking credibility. A dismissive trait I'm sure John Foxx of Ultravox once referred to as 'punk Stalinism.' Despite my musical snobbery and the fact stadium rock is a prime candidate for anathema to my tastes, the alcohol is making INXS danceable. The chlorpromazine in my bloodstream disagrees.

My meds have been spending all night tightening their straightjacket. I try moving my hands. Even my fingers. They're locked by my side. It's the weirdest sensation. This must be how a spider's prey feels after being injected with venom and shrouded in a web.

Raising her eyebrows my partner glances at her pal. Her friend mouths something at Alex, fires me the type of look reserved for shoe inspection after trodding on dog shit. The pair disengage and head deeper into the knot of bodies, there to be pounced upon by another pair of roving males; neither of whom has included antipsychotic drugs in their night's intake.

Grasping my collar, Alex marches me back. Those in the vicinity recognise the body language. Nightclub punch-ups have been a regular occurrence since the protagonists wore drape jackets and quiffs. Dancers back away, anticipating the first blow. I pre-empt it. By a gut reaction. I throw up over him.

No warning is given. No drawn-out minutes of nausea. I just gawk at him. Blink a couple of times. Then my stomach explodes.

I hose his choleric features, his white shirt, his trousers, his buckled shoes, and a three-foot radius around him. I splatter various gobsmacked by-dancers.

Alex grabs my arm and leads me from the floor. A bouncer spots the commotion. He looks like a Neanderthal in a suit. He makes his way over in the manner of a bull homing in on a flashing red neon sign. Alex steps in front and murmurs something. Points at me. I wait for the apoplectic bouncer to brush him aside like a fly. Instead, he nods. His expression relaxes. He gives me a thumbs-up.

Alex faces me and says he's going to get cleaned. But he told the bouncer the score, namedropping Andy. When I shrug, he elaborates. He explained I'm an outpatient from the Andrew Duncan Clinic and I've suffered a severe reaction to my meds. He adds the bouncer is getting the door staff to order a Joe Baksi.

My jaw hits the deck as this heavyset guy reaches for a walkie-talkie that must have summoned reinforcements during countless brawls. Chewing gum, he relates the message, winks at me.

A few glances are cast towards the bouncer hovering by the wasted-looking guy before everyone's attention returns to 'Theme from S'Express' and the mating ritual.

*

I ask the cab driver to drop me on Slateford Road, allowing a five-minute stroll through the cool night. I become aware of booming music. It's quarter to three in the morning but this sounds like a raucous house party is in full flow. Tracing the noise to its source, I find myself staggering to a tenement's top floor. Puffing from the inevitable 20+ tab accompaniment to a night's serious drinking, I arrive at the landing, stumbling into a neighbour's pot plant and kicking earth everywhere.

I shove my left hand into my jacket, thinking of the scene in *The Godfather* when Michael Corleone orders a hospital visitor to disguise himself as a bodyguard, demanding he shoves a hand inside a jacket to clutch an invisible gun. I'm grasping a pretend quarter bottle of vodka. My free hand rattles the letterbox. The door swings open.

A middle-aged woman gazes at me like a lab technician scrutinising an unknown substance manifesting on a slide. I claim to have met John along at The Mill earlier, who said I should drop by. When she remains impassive, I suggest it wasn't John. Jim?

She stays poker-faced. I enquire if this is *the* party. She replies this is *the* party for her grandson's 18th. Reinforcements muster behind. Someone turns the music down. My bravado evaporates. I recover enough to conjure an escape route. I enquire if this is Shandon Crescent? When she tells me Shandon *Street*, I grin and about turn, crunching through the earth from the disturbed plant pot.

The door slams. If she was peeping through the spyhole she would've witnessed me tug out the non-existent bottle, uncap it, take a slug, then grimace.

39

Terminal

June 1988

Every morning Mum provides my alarm call, rapping on the door then bustling into my room with a tray of tea, toast, and job adverts from newspapers scissored into neat rectangles. While I'm keen to get back into the labour force, I'm carrying so much more baggage than most applicants.

As she hands them the tray, she suggests I phone the temp agency and find out if there are any openings. After watching her exit, I study each vacancy between mouthfuls. The bedroom door opens again and she hands over the portable phone.

After breakfast, I call the agency. They tell me there's an opening tomorrow at the Scottish Equitable head office. I picture the building. It's on St Andrew Square, overlooking the Traveller's Tryst. Just like old times.

*

The terminal display seems unfathomable as crop circles. An elaborate spreadsheet partitions figures into columns, sub-totals, carry-forwards, and grand totals. In the top corner, the cursor blinks, demanding to be set off on some purposeful voyage through this arithmetical morass.

Sunlight filters through the grubby windows from St Andrew Square. I worked in the office block on the other side of the bus station before my breakdown. The employment agency kept me on their books, although I wonder if this instigated heated debates among the office staff about my employability. This temp job is my first gainful employment in over eight months.

This is my third day at this clerical post, seconded to the Scottish Equitable Insurance Company. It took less than five minutes to demonstrate my main task, something to do with amending policy records.

Although I'm no longer partying like I was at the previous job, popping down to the Traveller's Tryst at the drop of a hat, I've found it hard to resist a lunchtime drink. Instead of cramming in several pints with chasers, I've been making my way to The Highwayman in the middle of the bus depot for a plate of lasagne washed down with a solitary pint.

By two in the afternoon I'm staring into this VDU like a goldfish, eyelids transformed to lead. The white numerals against the shimmering green background become hieroglyphics, performing zany dances. The atmosphere of tap-tapping keyboards, trilling phones, and muted conversations recedes into waves crashing on a shore. Reverting decades, I'm on the beach at Coldingham Bay with my cousin Ross and our English mate, Jol. Dashing in and out of the crashing waves. Taunting them like three little King Canutes.

A voice demands to know if I'm sleeping. Sitting bolt upright I see Kirsty glaring across the desks. She was the one assigned to show me the ropes between ten past and quarter past nine on Monday morning. I guess she's around 21, with a neat perm, a turned-up nose, and an engagement ring.

Looking down at the keyboard, and down that pug nose at my earrings and post-punk spikes, she explained everything to me with all the emotion of an Auschwitz guard on a train platform ordering prisoners which queue to join. Now her expression is so indignant she might as well have substituted 'sleeping' with 'masturbating'.

I mention needing an early night. Lips pursed, she shakes her head. Students, she murmurs, before nodding at the pile of forms on my desk. Once I've finished inputting the data from that screed, I've not to sit there staring into space, or catching up on my sleep. I've to ask her for the next batch of forms.

Yesterday she took me into a store cupboard, pointed to piles of A4 sheets, like those improbable stacks of dirty dollar bills you see in mobster movies. I was told to count these into batches of 50. Not 49 or 51. 50. These were then to be fixed together with tiny bulldog clips. Performing this task beneath the humming striplights I felt like the central character in a Franz Kafka short story. Mind drifting, I mused about my life being the other way round. I imagined my Higher History periods at Tynecastle High consisting of counting sheets into batches. Then being paid a salary for writing essays about how the Jacobite defeat at Culloden presaged the ethnic cleansing of Scotland's Highlands, the suppression of our Gaelic culture, and the Caledonian diaspora.

I give the computer screen my undivided attention.

*

Mum and Dad are visiting their friends the Joliffes in Middlesbrough. They first met on holiday in St Abbs in 1964 and reunite there every summer. Their son, another Mark, Jol to Anne and I, a motorcycle and heavy metal fanatic, roadie and carpenter, is my longest-standing mate. We've shared so many adventures, from the days of 'best man falls' on Coldingham Bay's towering dunes, to riotous drinking sessions culminating in carryouts and campfires beneath the jaw-dropping majesty of the starscape above the North Sea untainted by light pollution.

I'll always be indebted to Jol for introducing me to his cassettes of The Sex Pistols, The Stranglers and The Jam one holiday when we were still school kids, instigating the seachange in my musical tastes that would later be augmented by my mate Ross in Edinburgh, one of the first Tynecastle pupils to 'turn punk,' and invent an alter-ego, Arthur Accident. I look forward to catching up with Jol again this August.

I took advantage of their jaunt down the A1 by phoning the agency to lie about extreme food poisoning. So I've been bingeing on videos, catching up on favourite LPs and cassettes. Last night I got wrecked at Grum's Haymarket flat before embarking on a West End pub crawl.

Waking up to another hangover, I make myself a pot of tea, several butter-drenched toast slices, then decide to phone in again. The stomach upset is persisting.

Around ten minutes after phoning the agency, the phone goes. It's Gail, one of the managers. She passes on a message from a Steven Fleming – no relation – some personnel manager from their client. They're letting me go. This has got nothing to do with my recent absences. The work I was contracted to do has pretty much dried up. The moment anything else crops up, she'll be sure to call.

I glare at the loose change that spilt everywhere when I stumbled from my jeans in the small hours after drinking in L'Attache until closing time. The price of punching another gaping hole in my CV.

40

Nikki

Digging into my carryout I hand over a tin of Strongbow, flip one for myself, and ask Bill how many of his mates have arrived. Not many yet, he replies, winking, before nodding towards the living room. I've to make myself at home; he's just popping to the loo.

I pause by the door. Never the most confident social being, I avoid being forced into company with strangers. At primary, I boycotted playground breaks for the first week, just me in the class with Mrs Marwick, doing a jigsaw (featuring an Alsatian dog, as I recall). While everyone else was running around and emptying their lungs at Cubs, Scouts, then youth clubs, I'd be hovering on the periphery. Mixing with people from other offices at training courses or seminars always raised my blood pressure. My nightmarish experience in my early teens had dashed any hope of that reticence fading into adolescence.

My innate diffidence was tested when the agency promoted me to a supervisor earlier in the year. I found myself having to bark at a table of 15 adults often behaving no better than nursery kids. Like The Speaker at Westminster. Except instead of *order, order*, I'd hiss, *could you please keep the noise down?* If that didn't work, I'd repeat my demand, my frayed nerves condensing this to, *fucking zip it for a bit, guys?* Detonating an F-bomb usually worked. For a few minutes. Although I could sympathise with lapsing into verbose banter during hours of clerical drudgery because I'd been there.

The agency manager took me aside with a whispered warning: only the supervisors would survive the next round of redundancies. Attempting to adopt a shell of assertiveness seemed a small price to pay for keeping my job. That's all so academic, given the water that has since flooded under the bridge.

I feel my heart thundering. Who'd be on the other side of this door, listening to The Waterboys blasting from Bill's record player? When he phoned earlier, I asked who else he'd invited. He replied *a few friends* before giving directions to his Tollcross flat. Now I wonder if these few friends will be from the outside world, or other outpatients? Would this gathering be a ward meeting with tinnies instead of tablets?

'The Whole of the Moon' fades into the next track on *This Is The Sea*, the stabbing piano intro to 'Spirit.' I neck several gulps of cider. Seizing the handle, I fail to stifle a belch of rutting elephant seal proportions. Embarrassment envelops me as I blunder in. There's no one else in the room.

Nodding to Mike Scott's soulful voice, I sit on the thread-bare couch. I met Mike once, in a pub in Ayr, when I spent the weekend at Tom's parents. Although Mike is Edinburgh-born, he moved to Ayr aged 12. To Tom, he was just a boy he knew from school who'd gone on to share a path familiar to many 1960s kids, myself included, embracing the punk scene in their mid-teens.

Mike published his own 'zine, *Jungleland*, subtitled 'Ayr's first rock 'n' roll fanzine,' named after a Bruce Springsteen song. But also inspired by his childhood in Clermiston on Edinburgh's west side. 'Welcome to Jungleland,' was graffitied onto a wall, signposting the territorial boundary of the local street gang, Young Clerrie Jungle.

Like so many of his peers, his writing fixated on The Clash and The Sex Pistols but also paid homage to earlier innovators like John Cale, Lou Reed, and Patti Smith (to whom The Waterboys' first single, 'A Girl Called Johnny,' was a tribute).

He returned to the capital in 1977 to study English Lit at Edinburgh University, just as the capital's punk scene was gathering momentum, forming a power-pop band, Another Pretty Face with a fellow Ayr ex-pat, John Caldwell, on guitar.

Bringing my musings around in a complete circle, I recall John's younger brother, Bruce who once played in my band, Desperation A.M. First introducing himself to us as 'Coddy,' his audition was a note-perfect rendition of '2-4-6-8 Motor-way,' by the Tom Robinson Band.

More circles: our bassist, Ross, saw the Tom Robinson Band the first time they played Edinburgh, in September 1978, after going along to catch their support band, Stiff Little Fingers. He met the Belfast punks in the Odeon foyer, got their autographs. Another Pretty Face supported Stiff Little Fingers on tour two years later after signing with Virgin. Between Another Pretty Face and The Waterboys came the short-lived Funhouse, named after The Stooges' riotous second album and described by Mike as sounding *similar to a jumbo jet flying on one engine.*

Anyone's life can consist of circles. It's also akin to joining dots, forming intriguing bigger pictures you're only aware of once when isolated dots are linked.

The next track, 'The Pan Within,' mellow and medium-paced, enables me to hear the stair buzzer, then a minute or so later, a timid knock at the front door.

Bill enters the room, accompanied by a short guy with carrot-coloured hair and thick-lensed glasses who stares into the carpet when Bill introduces him as Simon. Simon presents me with the limpest handshake I've ever encountered.

Sitting cross-legged, Bill tugs from a pencil-thin roll-up while sipping from the beaker he has decanted red wine into. As we chat, Simon just nods. If I thought I was introverted, he takes bashfulness to new depths, his cheeks flaring in the aftermath of his mumbled one-word responses to any of the questions we fire at him to try and coax him into the conversation. But he seems happy enough. And who am I to judge?

When I first met Bill on Ward 5, he was bubbly, skating along the upside of his schizophrenia, just back from a session in

The Canny Man's. We clicked. Now I muse that mates tend to meet through common interests. Hobbies. A love of football. A passion for music. Perhaps in a bar or club under the influence of alcohol, speed, weed, etc. Our common denominator is mental illness. A manic depressive and two schizophrenics whose initial introductions occurred under the influence of loxitane, thiothixene, stelazine, mellaril, chlorpromazine, etc.

In yet another coincidence, Ayr also happens to be Bill's home town. He begins chatting about the football. Like so many living within the Old Firm tractor beam, he isn't interested in his local team, Ayr United, but is a fervent Rangers supporter. He told me he was brought up Roman Catholic, making him one of the bluenose minority forced to adopt selective hearing during the incessant terracing bigotry, although this apparent contradiction is now less noteworthy.

Graeme Souness was appointed manager last year, accepting the role on the understanding that, despite decades of the club's heinous rule about never signing Catholics, the religious persuasion of his prospective new players was to be as relevant as the colour of their stools.

Perhaps this noble attempt to counter decades of institutionalised prejudice has had as much impact on the core of their support as King Canute's attempt to alter the tidal currents of the North Sea. But anything is better than nothing.

Sectarianism, Scotland and Northern Ireland's version of South Africa's apartheid, or the former Confederate States' segregated buses, was the source of a disproportionate amount of beatings in Bill's youth. A crucifix necklace draped over a royal blue shirt was liable to provoke confusion and violence from morons on both sides.

When I ask Bill where all his other guests are, he admits there's only one more coming, whom he invited just to meet me, and who he then describes as five-eight, slim, brown eyes, short dark hair – punky, green streaks in it last week – and a great sense of humour. Fucking mad as a fish.

Simon adds this girl, Nikki, has nice jugs, although the effort of squeezing out so many syllables at once makes his ruddy cheeks appear to be coming close to boiling point. Chuckling, I sip more cider, and when Bill's intercom buzzes, my heart skips. I feel like a teenager in a youth club.

Nikki is vivacious. We hit it off straight away. Whenever I wind her up or direct harmless banter about Simon's shyness – a subject I can excel at after being on the receiving end of similar gibes for years – she guffaws. And she's tactile, nudging me to emphasise punchlines.

As the evening wears on, the four of us are guzzling so much booze the binliner containing the empties looks like it's concealing a misshapen body. I've been drinking half of each lager can, topping up with cider, as well as shifting large vodka and lemonades. Bill, Simon, and I appear to be on a self-destructive protest against the warnings to psychiatric outpatients about mixing meds and alcohol. Nikki is keeping pace.

As records conclude, Nikki and I roar requests. Bill's haphazard filing system would've struck a chord with John Peel, instigating digging into a large holdall crammed with cassettes, or poring over titles of albums and singles jammed into a small bookcase. Twice he prompts an alarming avalanche of vinyl onto the floor.

Our host takes pride that his furious rummaging usually results in that particular song being uncovered, everything from the topsoil unearthing of Motown, Squeeze, The Jackson 5, or James Brown, to the much deeper mining required to dig out some of my suggestions, such as Ultravox! – the exclamation mark indicating John Foxx was still the vocalist.

Nikki jokes that Bill's music collection is so eclectic because of his schizophrenia. Each of his personalities has individual tastes.

Whatever is played, we all dance to it. Across the floor, over the coach. The neighbours must assume a party is in full flow and wondered why they haven't heard more than three guests tramping up the stairwell. Nikki asks Bill if he's got any Gap Band and my heart soars when he pops on 'Burn Rubber On Me.'

I'm transported to the Hoochie Coochie Club, freaking out to this with my mate Colin Marshall, a psychobilly who I met through my friends Harry and Louise. At the time, all three were Rudolf Steiner pupils. As we stomp along to this funk classic, I'm thinking this is one of my best nights out since long before my hospitalisation.

When Simon jumps from the settee, he stumbles to the floor headfirst, Bill tripping over him. As they cackle in a drunken heap, neither in any great rush to extricate themselves, Nikki wraps her arms around my waist and launches her lips into mine. We neck, the music soaring, the room spinning, and when we break off she stares into my eyes and announces she's going to be sick.

*

As the cab trundles back towards town, Nikki shivers, pecks my cheek and mentions putting on the kettle. I take in the location. Murdoch Terrace, just up from the bakers run by the Lawrences from Shandon – I occasionally drank with their eldest lad, Neil, a Stranglers fan, in the Nirvana Hotel.

We enter a ground floor flat on a modern block next to Victorian tenements and I follow the seat of her ripped 501s. Inside she indicates a settee. She heads out to the kitchen.

Running water, a cupboard door, a fridge slamming. I hope her stomach has settled. When we kissed in the taxi I could taste toothpaste.

The door opens. A woman enters smoking a menthol ciga-rette. Maybe in her 40s. She almost misses her chair. Chuckles. Winking, she goes: *ssssssh!*

She's Carol. Nikki's mum. I tell her I'm a friend. When Carol asks if I mean, *boy*friend, I give an embarrassed shrug but nod. She thanks me for seeing Nikki home. They still worry about her. She was a wild teenager. Would go out with guys with mohawks. Multiple piercings.

I snigger at that, admitting I was into the punk thing, but way back. My concession to any notion of 'punk fashion' was straight-leg trousers, taken in by my mum. School blazers, customised with badges, spraypaint. Sometimes a homemade armband. By the time you'd see squads of 'punks' in identikit mail order uniforms, I'd drifted on to Gang of Four. Bauhaus. Cabaret Voltaire. Human League. Heaven 17.

Carol looks alarmed, as if I've started speaking in tongues. Stubbing out her fag, she heaves herself out of her armchair and shuffles through to the kitchen. Nikki and her mum laugh.

After a long sexual drought, I feel I've come up trumps. I accept alcohol is playing a part in my rapture but I do like Nikki. We'd so much to talk about in such a few hours, I feel a genuine connection. I've been admiring her curvy figure all night, hoping it won't just be wishful thinking for sex to be an intense extrapolation of her sparkling personality.

Down the corridor I glimpse her in a *London Calling* T-shirt and briefs, tugging on a cigarette, darting into the bathroom's glazed door. How liberal is her mother? Perhaps she doesn't condone her daughter bringing partners home because it's better than her former wild child *not* coming home.

I squint at my watch. Almost quarter past two. Carol appears with a tray containing steaming coffee, a milk jug, sugar bowl. She wishes me goodnight. Exits. Watching her stagger down the hall, I anticipate Nikki exiting the bathroom, beckoning. My eyes flicker. I blink away the sleep but the couch feels like a raft drifting on lugubrious currents.

*

The VHS player's display has fast-forwarded to 05:38. I note the untouched coffee, milk forming a ring around its surface. Then I notice the man staring at me. This has a sobering effect. His combover accentuates his baldness. His stare is unflinching, as if I'm a Texan criminal and he's about to administer the lethal injection. Sucking from a cigarette, he puffs the acrid cloud over me, then enquires who the fuck I am.

Coming to, I bluster, I'm a friend of Nikki's.

Nicola, he corrects me.

Aye, I respond, murmuring she was going to make me a nightcap.

Glaring at the clock on the wall, he stands, jerking a thumb towards the door. I get to my feet, wobbling. He reaches out, nudges me down the hall. When I open the door, he asks if I'm a friend of Bill's. Is his abrupt manner at discovering a stranger in his living room thawing?

I answer I'm a good mate of Bill's. Mark. We met in hospital. I reach out to shake his hand. But he shoves me over the doorstep and snarls his daughter has always mixed with weirdos. He knows all about Bill. In and out the funny farm. They seem to let us out that place at the drop of a fucking hat. Not wanting Nicola hanging out with another daftie who might hear a voice ordering him to stab the poor lass. You read about that in the papers.

He slams the door hard enough to wake everyone in the block.

41

Jags

July 1988

While much of Scotland is tuning in to see if Pat Cash can emulate last year's surprise Men's Singles trophy at Wimbledon, I'm making the brisk 20-minute stroll into Morningside. Passing the leafy streets and sprawling mansions I glimpse green courts on TVs, imagine plummy voices congratulating winning passes.

I'm apprehensive but relieved this is so far removed from the time I made this same journey secured inside an ambulance. Crossing the hospital car park, a teenage lad is being escorted towards the shops by a nurse I recognise. In this cyclical system, he's a few laps behind.

In Ward 5 I nod at familiar faces. Bryan waves at me then disappears into the pharmacy. Minutes later he's ushering me towards a treatment room, asking how things are going on the outside. All good, I reply.

Unlocking the door, he gestures towards the couch with an exaggerated sweep of his hand, announcing my carriage awaits. Lying face down, I unbuckle my jeans, squirming while easing them past my thighs. I feel an icy touch as my right buttock is smeared with a freezing gel. In my peripheral vision, I see him preparing the syringe and tense. Impersonating Kenneth Williams, he says, *just a little prick, matron*. Although he cracks this same joke every time, I indulge him with a snigger, jolting as the needle pierces flesh.

This is my depot injection: antipsychotic medication suspended in vegetable oil to allow a gradual release, pre-empting regular oral medication. Another step along the long road to good health.

42

Bloods

August 1988

Strolling by the Union Canal, I cross the aqueduct above the railway. To my right, the line heads northwards towards Gorgie. Following the direction of the tracks for a few hundred yards I make out the two pipes traversing the steep embankment.

The railway was our favourite playground as kids. Maintenance workers often told us we were trespassing when they caught us dodging around shunters parked on sidings, issuing the equivalent of red cards: jotting our names and addresses in notebooks. For primary school kids, we got quite creative at conjuring ridiculous noms-de-plume.

We also delighted in crossing the wider of those pipes like demented tight-rope walkers, stabbing our middle fingers at the Grim Reaper. From this perspective, the distance to the sleepers far below is terrifying. My hangover exacerbates a sense of shock delayed by several decades.

To my left, a moorhen cleaves the canal's murky surface. Against the sunlight, the waterfowl appears to be swimming into flames. I smile at further reckless indifference to danger. But the light also bores into my pounding head. Last night Alex and I ended up in L'Attache until 1 a.m.

My recollections are distilled into muddy snapshots. Chatting-up numerous women, each of whom would see through my superficial charm and melt into the background. Roaring conversations with Alex about the music of our youth being so much better than the crap spilling from jukeboxes while knowing full well this is an argument destined to be repeated by subsequent generations *ad infinitum*. Some effusive folk band. An argument involving a guy wearing an Ireland rugby top and two mouth breathers calling him a fenian, a disturbance Alex and I got involved in.

I explained the Irish rugby colours represent *all* Ireland, Dublin to Belfast, Baile Áth Cliath to the Shankill Road, a point Alex underscored by chinning one of the WASP supremacists. Myself on sky blue helmet mode again later, separating Alex from another drunken prick who elbowed his way in front of two shivering young lassies at the Rutland taxi rank. Losing him outside Dario's. Somehow ending up arm-in-arm with an attractive redhead, a nurse, who reminded me of Carol Decker.

I recall telling her as much but provoking a rant against how shite T'Pau were compared to Guns N' Roses. We chatted for an age inside the foyer of the Florence Nightingale nursing home next to the Infirmary. I remember snogging beneath a cupola, the pale dawn filtering in, before a doorman appeared and ushered me outside to commence the long hike home. When I lit my final tab while staggering along the Shandon Colonies, I clocked the all-too-familiar sight of a name and number scrawled in eyeliner on my fag packet already reduced to a smudge.

I march up the path by the Meggetland bridge which served as a boundary during childhood forays into enemy territory. Not as in gangland but in the fantasy world my mates and I created.

Our imaginations conjured everyone from redcoats and Daleks to Nazis from *Commando* comics. Lurking amongst the undergrowth we crawled through, your pulse would quicken as you anticipated carving open a hapless German sentry's throat with your pretend knife before launching invisible grenades. That we were allowed to embark on these missions at such a distance from home seems incredible, although our parents had no reason to suspect we'd ventured any further than Harrison Park for a kickabout.

Further up Colinton Road, I lurch into my GP's surgery. In the waiting room, toddlers seem to be vandalising the box of toys rather than playing with anything. Seizing a *National Geographic*, I skim Midway Atoll shipwrecks where fish of every hue explore the graveyards of American and Japanese sailors. I glance at bored Scottish goldfish bobbing amongst the lemonade bubbles of their aquarium.

I'm relieved when Dr Patterson pokes his head around the door to summon me for my check-up. Inside his surgery, his first question is how my mental health has been. Although my reply of feeling 'back to normal' is so subjective, he seems more satisfied by my ability to articulate this, compared to the volatile behaviour highlighted in the file spread over his desk.

We chat about everything from my appetite to job searches. I tell him the latter is a constant turnover of applications and rejection letters, but I remain optimistic. Nodding at that, he concludes he's over the moon I've recovered from what he refers to as my 'awful wobble,' and will now undertake a routine physical examination.

He'll start by assessing my weight. I concede I've put on stones during all the inertia over the past year. He cautions that all the antipsychotic drugs I've been taking will also have impacted my metabolism. He wants to gauge my blood pressure, then take a blood sample because my medication can also impair renal function.

After assessing the blood pressure, he produces the rubber tourniquet and affixes it to my arm. Tapping a vein, he pokes the needle home, draws blood into the syringe. His reaction to the liquid filling the Perspex container is shock, giving way to amusement. He does aim a stare over the bows of his spectacle rims, reminding me I shouldn't be mixing excessive doses of alcohol with my meds.

I watch him labelling the phial containing the sample. It looks identical to the Pernod and blackcurrants I was necking a few hours ago.

43

Edinburgh Men

April 1989

The second day of my admin assistant job in the Scottish Record Office isn't progressing well. Arriving at work with a hangover from Hell, I struggle on until the 10 a.m. tea break, at which point I slink through the office side door, head around the corner, and clamber up the stairs to the Penny Black.

Like many pubs with extended opening hours, the bar is already three deep. A postie is accompanying 'Suspicious Minds,' on the jukebox; so off-key The King must be spinning like a lathe in his Graceland tomb. After he tumbles backwards from his barstool, I help to heave him up, then step in and order a double Jack Daniels and lemonade. This helps to soothe the vicious headache, but when I return to the office all I can think of is catching some shuteye. So I head into a toilet. I consult my watch. 10.25 a.m. My eyes waver shut.

There is an emphatic knock on the cubicle door. Flustered, I notice the time. 11.10 a.m. I recognise my line manager, Adrian's voice. He says they've been looking around the office for me but sounds concerned rather than annoyed.

Adrian is a jovial 40-something whose moustache and ruddy cheeks put me in mind of Captain Pugwash, although he prefers tank-tops to skulls and crossbones. I explain I was feeling queasy, but this seems to be passing.

If I'm unwell there's no point forcing myself to hang around. There are a few bugs doing the rounds. So he suggests I head home, phone in tomorrow with an update. I inject my voice with enough despondency to remain this side of over-acting, agreeing that shaking off my bug would be preferable to passing it on.

I wait until the outside door slams before clambering to my feet, punching the air like a Tartan Army footsoldier when Archie Gemmill caressed the ball past Jan Jongbloed in Argentina. Grasping my coat, I head outside into glorious sun-shine, ducking into The Guildford Arms. Now confident my stomach has settled enough, I order a pint. As I watch the lager settling I'm aware of another patron ordering a lager and a whisky chaser in a nasal Mancunian tone. I recognise the voice straight away.

I'm transported back to my teenage bedroom, fingers poised on my Hi-Fi cassette deck's play/record buttons when John Peel announced the next track in the latest session by The Fall. I turn to my side. In a day where each weird event is being superseded, my boss gifting me a sickie has just been trumped by discovering myself standing beside Mark E Smith, English post-punk legend, in an Edinburgh city-centre pub. Although starstruck, I manage to hold it together long enough to play it cool, paying for my pint, savouring the first few mouthfuls. I turn to him. *Mark Smith?*

He affirms this fact, shoving a hand out. I introduce myself, shaking the digits responsible for scribing some of the most caustic urban poetry to have emanated from these islands. I know he's a City fan but recall an interview where he professed his admiration of George Best's mercurial abilities. I mention the Guildford was one of his favoured bars after he signed for the Hibs in 1979. Often en route to Easter Road.

Mark casts up the story of his temporary sacking for embarking on a binge with the visiting French rugby team. Although he got his Northern Ireland caps no matter his club form, Best always championed a United Ireland team. Toasting that observation, we chink glasses.

I ask what's brought him to Edinburgh, am bowled over to learn he's living in the New Town. Despite journalistic cliches about him being a 'difficult interviewee,' his conversation is engaging. And scattershot, switching topics at a dizzying pace.

He loves the Malt Whisky Society down in Leith. Then he reveals he dropped by the war memorial on the Mound earlier today on his travels. Asks if I know it. I can picture the statue of a kilted soldier opposite Misty's on the Mound. He explains it's dedicated to Black Watch who died in the Boer War. His father, Jack served in the regiment in World War 2.

I tell him about my mum's grandad, William Ballantyne. He served in the Boer War. Promoted to a corporal. Twelve years later, some fuckwit placed a white feather inside his jacket, compelling him to volunteer again, although he was in his 30s by then. He joined the Black Watch. After three weeks in France, he was killed. April 16th 1915. Left a wife with six kids, decades before social security, consigned to poverty in Edinburgh's South Side. Their mother was out so my grannie read the official telegram to her siblings. She'd just turned 12.

Topping up last night's alcohol loosens my tongue. One of my happiest memories of Grannie surfaces. I describe her listening to a demo tape of my band at a family party, standing up in front of everyone and jigging along to the music on her own – the oldest post-punk in Scotland.

But I decide not to labour the band thing. Mark must be sick to the back teeth of being pestered by young fans extolling their own groups. Claiming The Fall as an influence, or using the term 'post punk' would guarantee to set those teeth on edge. Unless you were in the position of being cited as the next Can or Captain Beefheart, his enthusiasm would be on a par with you describing lift muzak.

I lapse into fanboy mode. There are so many questions I want to blurt out, one for every Blue Tack morsel I once poked into the cuttings from *Sounds* and *NME* about The Fall to adorn every spare inch of one bedroom wall. I tell him how much I loved *Live At The Witch Trials*. When Dave McCullough reviewed it in *Sounds* he referred to 'Industrial Estate' as *perhaps the ultimate punk song*.

He baulks at pigeon-holing The Fall as a punk band, before telling me it was that album's tenth anniversary a few weeks back. By the time it was released, Bramah and Burns, his lead guitarist and drummer, had both fucked off, leaving him the sole original member. Smiling at that, he downs his whisky. I realise the faux-pas of fixating on their debut album. The Fall are the last band to wallow in nostalgia, with even die-hard fans often lucky to recognise more than a third of any set at a gig.

I profess my love for *This Nation's Saving Grace*, fast-forwarding to a previous occasion our paths crossed, although I doubt he'll remember. That album, their eighth, came out in September 1985. I saw The Fall a month later at Coasters, the venue once known as Clouds, the epicentre of the capital's live punk scene where I also saw them in February 1981.

I happened to have three of my latest short stories with me, folded into my jacket pocket, having intended to give them to my mate Kenny, Little Big Dig's new bassist. His compact, controlled but emphatic basslines truly anchored our music compared to our previous player, Colin, whose fretless style had been more fluid, improvisational, sometimes veering into jazz, more than occasionally inspired by the bong he'd clearly been hoovering a half hour before. Kenny was Steve Hanley to Colin's Jah Wobble. Each exhilarating in their own way.

Included amongst these stories was one entitled 'Legless in Gatsby's,' an account of the time I was barred from that pub, and which had just been published in my local community newspaper, *Gorgie Dalry Gazette*. Setting tongues wagging because of its uncensored F-word content.

After The Fall's set, I spotted Mark weaving into the club's cloakroom-cum-dressing room. A golden opportunity had presented itself. Emboldened by alcohol, I rapped on the door. The Hip Priest himself swung it open and was about to slam it in my face when I thrust the crumpled A4 sheets into his bemused grasp.

Some stories I've written, Mark. Check them out. You've always been an inspiration. You, James Kelman... Well. Just you and James Kelman.

Kelman? I've read some of his stories. Acid? About a guy falling into a vat of fucking acid in a factory? One paragraph long or something? Love that salt of the earth Scottish stuff. It's authentic. Totally fucking authentic. Hey, Craig. Give the lad a can.

There, in Coaster's nightclub, Mark E Smith accepted the tin of Carlsberg Special from guitarist Craig Scanlan and handed it to me. It felt like being presented with the Scottish Cup. A wink and the door closed. I flipped the tin open and toasted the moment of utter kudos.

Four weeks later, our manager's partner, Muriel interviewed Mark and his wife Brix after an appearance on *The Tube*. Muriel commented about their band's huge following, despite his seeming indifference to the limelight. He acknowledged his band's cult status, adding the people who followed The Fall were the *salt of the earth*, but *not the type to attack you in supermarkets*.

He went on to admit he rarely read fanmail and would only write back to those people he found interesting. Secretly,

I hoped his response to my fiction was in the post, although I suspected my stories ended up crumpled amongst the empty Carlsberg cans in the Coasters dressing room.

My memento took pride of place on the top shelf of the unit in my bedroom, above all my Fall records, until one day I noticed its absence. Assuming it was one of my dad's empties, Mum binned it.

One reason for flitting from Manchester might have been to escape being pestered in bars. So I decide a tactical retreat is in order, explaining I've just started working over the road. We might share pints in The Guildford again.

We chink glasses. I snatch mine from the bar and scuff over to a window seat, there to go over the endless possibilities of conversation topics I could've broached.

44

Glasgow Men

March 1990

Good evening. We are The Fall. We are a cool group, deadpans Mark E Smith to roaring acclaim. He glares into the Barrowlands crowd as Simon Wolstencroft launches into a thunderous drumbeat. A more danceable progression to their last album, *I Am Kurious Oranj*, the baggy rhythm gets the punters bouncing. When the *NME* reviewed their forthcoming album, *Extricate*, the headline was 'Fall's Gold,' also alluding to Madchester and The Stone Roses. They gave it 10/10.

For a fleeting moment, Smith catches my eye and I wonder if he'll recognise the guy who cornered him in an Edinburgh pub. But his gaze moves on, flitting over the rammed audience towards the chequered ceiling tiles.

I'm finding it hard to concentrate on anything. I'm now seeing two of him, as well as Martin Bramah, back on guitar 12 years after *Live At The Witch Trials*. Steve Hanley's disjointed bassline is pounding my rib cage, and the proximity of so many sweaty bodies is augmenting my discomfort.

Horror, error! squeals Smith. He's describing how I feel. After extricating myself from a plum position near the stage, I struggle through the weight of bodies, like a salmon facing falls. Finding the steps leading towards the bar, I hunker down. The Fall launch into a track from *Extricate*. 'The Littlest Rebel.'

Hemmed in by a forest of denim and black, the floor shifts. I stare at my Sambas, riding a wave of nausea. I wonder how I arrived here. The background music recedes into a distorted cacophony eating into the fuzziness inside my head. I just want to curl into a ball. And sleep. My eyes close.

I come to with a jolt. I've no idea where I am, or why I've woken amongst a throng of strangers. A mysterious liquid oozes down my neck. Someone thought it would be hilarious to tip their beer over the alcohol casualty. Paranoia consumes me. I gaze around but this only makes me even dizzier. Everyone is rooted to something going on in the distance. A hand reaches from the crowd, grasps my shoulder. *Mark! What in the name of fuck happened to you?*

It takes an age to focus. It's my buddy, Tom. He insists I was supposed to be in Bairds at eight and he waited fucking ages. Peering up, I take in his familiar features. It's been three years since Little Big Dig split and he moved to London. He phoned during the week. Up visiting his mum in Ayr, he suggested hooking up here.

I announce I've been on the piss since before nine in the morning and am cunted. He shakes his head. Bemoans the fucking state of me, and the miracle of me blagging my way by the bouncers. He tells me he's going to get the drinks in. When I demand a double voddie and coke he says he'll order a pint of fresh orange and lemonade, fuck all else.

He's gone. I listen to Smith. *I hear you Telephone Thing, listening in,* over a single-note bass riff that pulverises my guts. I try rewinding, piecing together the day's shattered jigsaw.

Breakfast consisted of vodka and orange. I decanted the liquor into a lemonade bottle which I forced down my neck on the Union Jack supporters' bus. Defying the law that outlaws attempting to enter Scottish football grounds under the influence of alcohol, I stumbled through the Love Street turnstiles and up the flight of stairs to the visitors' portion of the main terracing. Staggered over to the segregation barrier, singling out a pair of bemused Buddies fans wearing spectacles. They became *Joe 90 bastards* at intermittent stages of the game.

This idiotic bawling through the fence persisted until I became aware of a policeman near the touchline fixing me in his cross-hairs. So I zipped it until the final whistle, as per most of my boozy Saturday afternoons, blasé about the game's outcome.

Hitching a lift on the first Rangers bus I came across heading back into Glasgow, I jumped off at the lads' local. Throwing Löwenbräu down my neck, I contemplated visiting my Auntie Molly, whose Pollokshaws address was only a few blocks away, before lurching off to hose lager down the toilet.

Somehow I found my way to Queen Street Station and was refused service in the Clyde Bar. Sprawled on a bench outside I got chatting to a bunch of kids claiming to be ICF waiting to ambush Celtic fans returning from Dunfermline.

My mate Mike Sylvester – Silly – alighted from the next Edinburgh train. He stays along the road from my folks in Shandon, was in Anne's year at school, three years below. We're good mates, sharing musical tastes, going to gigs. In the punk days, we spent Saturday afternoons rifling through the vinyl in Bruce's, Virgin, Hot Licks, and The Other Record Shop. Now he couldn't mask how appalled he was at my dishevelment.

We taxied it to Barrowlands, the driver eyeballing me in his rear-view mirror, suspecting I was on the verge of coating the floor with vomit. We headed into the pub next door, Bairds, a shrine to Celtic, with wall-to-wall tricolours, team portraits, and Lisbon Lions pendants. Every so often I checked out the décor, lip curling like an Elvis impersonation. Two pints later my arm was wrapped around a stranger at the bar, insisting his club's achievements in 1967 made fans of every Scottish team proud. Every *British* team, since they were the first to lift the European Cup. Every team bar fucking one, he pointed out, winking.

Now the swaying sensation, so alarming a moment ago, seems more reassuring. I almost manage a grin. But this fades. Why this drunk, every other Saturday? Why Glasgow? When I twisted Dad's arm to take me to Easter Road and Jimmy O'Rourke or Alan Gordon rifled one in, my childhood heart would rupture. If Coisty scores now I tend to see his celebrations against a backdrop of 44 players and six officials, before squinting at both my watches to check how long before I can return to the nearest bar.

Today's trip to Paisley was a blur. Every supporters' bus has raucous teenagers occupying the upstairs back seats, although some of the Jack's younger team defected to the Hibs mob, Capital City Service. The remaining ones delight at my condition every other week, rolling up the aisle minutes before departure. This morning I paid one of them a fistful of coins for a one-skinner. They cackled like hyenas at my confusing a niccy buzz for the non-existent tarry.

Vodka for breakfast. Coffee breaks in the Penny Black and Buff's Club. Alcohol blending with lithium. Taking my antipsychotic drugs before every binge in case I forgot later; sometimes neglecting this precaution, then hovering bleary-eyed before the bathroom cabinet in the wee small hours, weighing up the risks of doubling the dose against the side effects of failing to take any meds; either decision adding paranoia about impairment of my kidney and liver functions to feeling awful the following day. The vicious circle. *Hair of the dog*. A stiff whisky or vodka always a preferable option to what Mum once described as the Craigentinny version of a stiff upper lip: Grandad 'tholing' his hangovers.

I struggle to remember who's just gone to the bar. Tom. This brings back pissed-up Little Big Dig practices. Weekends in the Hooch with the guys from the band. Necking snakebite after snakebite until I was lurching around the club as if I *had* been bitten by a cobra. Eyeballing Paul Haig, the original singer of Edinburgh post-punk legends Josef K as he exited the toilets, blowing a raspberry into his face for no other reason than jealousy he'd reached the stage of being a respected singer/songwriter, worthy of being interviewed on *The Tube* by Muriel Gray strolling around Greyfriar's Churchyard while I remained in one of the many bands scrabbling for recognition by sending demo tapes everywhere.

Also at the Hooch. Another beered-up regular from Shandon. Si. Psychobilly-turned-Hearts Boy. Embracing him like a long-lost buddy. Si, who went to Augys, bragging about a mate decking someone in the Wheatsheaf for wearing a Guinness T-shirt, *the fucking harp and everything*. I suggested this religious bigotry wasn't very Christian, to which Si took my breath away by stating his buddy wasn't Christian but *defo* Protestant. When I pointed out Guinness were a Protestant family he just shrugged before breaking into the British national anthem, its obsequious sentiment and thuggish right-wing undercurrents jarring with the cool vibes and joyous music enveloping everyone else: Frankie Goes To Hollywood, Screaming Nobodies, The Gap Band, Fire Engines, Pete Shelley, Grandmaster Melle Mel, Bronski Beat, Echo and the Bunnymen; or the affable dancefloor melees when the psychobillies piled on top of each other during The Meteors.

A whirlwind of chaotic incidents. Waiting for transport by Basin Street, this supporter's bus typifying these weekend outings more than any eventual match attendance. For most of the passengers, it *was* about following a club based 48 miles away, singing the players' praises, collecting the merchandise.

But for me, these excursions were almost detached from the actual football.

It was a temporary escape from 9 to 5 drudgery and an uncertain future courtesy of my medical history. I'd keep schtum about my first team – the Leith Celts or spoon-burners to most of the lads – and the posters and programmes I still revered. Even more closely-guarded secrets were my father being born in Monaghan, under the tricolour, and his brother having married a left-footer.

But every Saturday had become an alcohol-fuelled adventure. A bipolar mystery tour. It was about the camaraderie of 'the Jack,' with many of the more seasoned members just as likely to be rubbed up the wrong way by the weegie-accented supporters drinking beside them in bars the length and breadth of Scotland as any opposing fans.

One syllable short of camaraderie? Kamikaze. Some guys on that bus cultivated ferocious reputations. Len and Hutchie. Wester Hailes space cadets. Hiding their scarves to gain entry to 'the Shed' at Tynecastle before producing their colours and goading the home support for frenetic moments while awaiting the police escort, a performance earning grudged respect from the Hibs Boys they worked beside. Len returning to the bus after Old Firm encounters grinning like an excited kid, clutching green, white and orange scarves seized from opposing fans. *Scalps*, he'd add with his toothless grin.

One nadir of this hooliganism. Len and Hutchie hurling abuse at the Celtic supporters gathering outside Ryrie's waiting for their pick-up, a microcosm of the Old Firm lunacy bewildering tourists and West End shoppers. The Celtic bus arriving, filling up, taking off. Something arcing through the air. Glistening against the sunlight. A fleeting thing of beauty, captivating as Maradona weaving through the English defence at Estadio Azteca in Mexico City. Its speed, direction and trajectory towards the retreating coach judged to perfection, like the Ile Nastase aces shaving the line that would delight Mum watching Wimbledon. Except this moment was the antithesis of sport.

The bottle impacting the rear window, imploding against the Irish tricolour. A detonation that made your stomach churn, like watching the news footage of the Challenger's demise. The vehicle squealing to a halt. Furious guys in hooped shirts decanting, thinking twice as a mob of blue-bedecked nutters charged. A convoy of blues and twos swarming over from Torphicen Street police station, ushering the Celtic fans into the coach booked for the Jack. Disgruntled bluenoses cursing the window vandal while awaiting the replacement, knowing they'd miss a chunk of whatever game was the excuse for all this.

More madness. Big Rab, in my year at Tynecastle, so drunk it was an effort to stand, Hutchie clasping his belt while he pished out the bus doorway, bawling *'Follow, follow,'* the M8 roaring by at 80 miles-per-hour. Bumping into him in Platform One, slumped against a pillar to keep upright, a folk band leading the packed and sweaty clientele into rollicking choruses of 'The Wild Rover,' the rebellious exuberance flowing around him, the rock of ignorance, slurring his version of the chorus: *And it's Glasgow Rangers... God save our Queen... Glasgow Rangers FC...*

Or the ex-Scout flag I took to a league game against Hearts at Ibrox in February, masking taped with 'EDINBURGH UNION JACK RSC.' Entering Ryries long after the match, the pub rammed with French supporters drowning their sorrows after their 21-0 Six Nations drubbing at Murrayfield earlier, greeting the late surge of red, white and blue-bedecked Gallic buddies, then recoiling from the belligerent local accents and this unfamiliar flag for Scottish sporting events. The brief flowering then dousing of mistaken comradeship akin to Falls Road residents serving tea to the squaddies who arrived to protect their homes from being burned out by their Loyalist neighbours before polar opposite sentiments were ignited by Internment, the Ballymurphy Massacre, and Bloody Sunday; regurgitating memories of the Tans terrorising older relatives.

That interminable day's bingeing didn't even halt there and those colours ended up being brandished on the Buster Brown's dancefloor.

Drunken matadors. Could be a Fall song title. I fixate on Steve Hanley's hypnotic bass. Visualise Mark E Smith glowering into me. Salford tones dripping with scorn. Another remorseless wave of fatigue is drawing me into a fitful gouch. My head slumps. I'm spellbound by Smith's voice, grasping for it like a lifeline as I sink into a stupor until his scathing nasal drawl becomes the last thing I'm aware of. My intoxicated, slumbering mind perverting his language, his squeaky, serrated knife-edge vocalising conjures a hallucinatory Fall song...

Drunken matadors brandishing their butcher's aprons. Heathen matadors-uh. Extolling religion from a hellbound position-uh. Telling *Him* you *refuse* to love thy neighbour-uh. You *hate* thy neighbour. Pro-test-ant matadors-uh. Stomp jackboots, bang drums, wave flags. Drape the cunting bunting-uh. Dredge up the black poison of centuries-uh. Curious oranj-uh. *Curious oranj-uh.* William of *Oranj*, no mistresses-uh. Only Bentinck and Van Keppel. Pretty wigs for his courtiers-uh. English titles for his little Dutch boys-uh. Earl of Portland, Earl of Albermarle-uh. Three hundred years later, the *oranj* beat still crashing-uh. Still marching as to war, still crossing the Boyne-uh. And the Darian peasants starving. Scottish aliens starving-uh. Union of fucking crowns my arse-uh. C of E tips the balance, bloodies the Glencoe snow on Billy boy's orders-uh. Killing Times for Covenanters, for thousands of C of S swinging on gibbets-uh. Exiled as Caribbean slaves-uh. White crap whipped if it talks back. *Drunken matadors-uh.*

I snap out of it.

There's three members of the group who like to cut songs in half, y'know, Smith announces after a version of 'British People in Hot Weather' is curtailed. The drums and bass kick off into the jerky intro to 'Bremen Nacht' from *Frenz Experiment*. It sounds brilliant but I just want The Fall, whose every vinyl release clutters my record collection, and whose every John Peel session I've captured on cassette, to shut the fuck up. Then I can start worrying about finding Silly in this rammed audience, and how the pathetic bundle of smash remaining in my pockets is going to whisk me across Central Scotland.

45

Mad Dogs

May 1990

After completing my 12 months as a casual administrative assistant in the Scottish Record Office, I sat an interview for placement in a permanent post. Adrian gave some sage advice. *Whenever you get asked a question, Mark, look the interviewer square in the eye.*

The time came and I was called into the office on Waterloo Place to be grilled by three executive officers. Adrian's words rang in my ears. The chairperson seemed affable, introducing himself with a firm handshake before launching into his broadside of questions. I fixed him in my sights. His eyes were all over the place. Like James Galway. The 'Man with the Golden Flute,' who has sold millions of records. Who has an eye condition called *nystagmus*. Also known as 'dancing eyes.' To avoid his gyrating pupils, I spent the next 20 minutes staring at the tip of his nose. This must have done the trick because a week later I received a letter offering a permanent position – with the strict proviso this would be probationary due to my 'underlying health condition.'

I later discovered Adrian asked the others in my team what they thought of me staying on in the Record Office. A unanimous veto was applied. The gist of their argument was my inclination to join the messengers in spending coffee breaks in the Penny Black or the Buff's Club, with forays to the bookies, rather than sitting in the coffee lounge reading *The Sun* or discussing last night's soaps. Instead, my permanent post, with its five-year probationary health clause, would commence with a Scottish Courts department, the Accountant in Bankruptcy, located in Meldrum House in the West End.

Living up to my 'reputation', my last day was marked by an extended lunch hour in the Penny Black drinking Southern Comfort and lemonades from noon until 3 p.m. I made a brief return to the office where I risked incurring the wrath of the Keeper of the Records by staggering into the main library, housed in an ornate Georgian room nicknamed the Dome, sparking up a Marlboro, attempting to chat up an attractive legal assistant, before flaking out over a desk.

*

I'm settling into a new department where most of my colleagues are also this side of 30. The office is far from the suited and tied bank or insurance environments I've experienced. The civil service has no strict dress code and when you pop down to grab files from the lektreivers you're assailed with Simon Bates, then Steve Wright on Radio 1.

This Friday lunchtime involves cheese toasties washed down with Stella Artois and double vodka and tonic chasers in Buskers. I'm back in the office by 2.35 p.m., seated in a toilet cubicle, tugging on my last tab. Fumbling inside my jeans I come across a dowt from a oneskinner. Sparking this, I get enough for a couple of draws before someone barges into the toilets, invoking a coughing fit as I karate chop the hash cloud lurking like a mischievous genie. Shuffling back to my desk, I stash fat awkward files into drawers. When my phone trills, I duck to my shoelaces until a colleague picks up.

The consensus is First Editions will be the kick-off point again. The happy 'hour' lasts from 5 p.m. until 7 p.m. I jot down the names of everyone to invite via an email string. Watching the wall clock creeping towards 4 p.m. is the slowest point of the entire week. There will be 15 of us at the start, although experience dictates this number will be thinned out by the natural attrition of a boozy Friday night in Edinburgh's city centre.

Ages range from Alison, a 17-year-old Fifer, to myself, the elder statesman at 27. Although Alison's a weekend raver, her Walkman reverberating with techno, she's not averse to pub crawls. Her boyfriend, John is an administrative officer in my team, one notch up the pecking order from me. Originally from Broughty Ferry, his main passions are lager, Ska, and Dundee United. When he was showing me the ropes on my first day, he was sporting a black eye, courtesy of a stramash with Dundee fans after the recent derby. Alison confided she suspected it happened at squash.

Chris is here until he resumes Uni after the summer. Alison has christened him Woodstock because of his long hair and beard, and his fondness for lunchtime toking along the nearby Water of Leith walkway. He also practices yoga in the staff canteen, bemusing the Inland Revenue staff who share our building.

Nina is another temp, younger than me, but we get on well. As we're opening the mail together we chat about shared musical tastes or wind each other up, often continuing these discussions in Buskers or The Ainslie, our frequent sanctuaries two minutes from the office.

When the time comes, the gang scuffs down the stairs into Buskers for a couple of rounds before heading along Drumsheugh Gardens, making for St Mary's Cathedral's steeples. Although it's near Haymarket station, First Editions is on the opposite side of the busy intersection. It's part of the West End Hotel, so it doesn't attract the usual flow of itinerants, jakeys and sectarian-minded football fans who often gravitate around station pubs. The first customers, we spread around tables before the video jukebox and widescreen TV.

Awaiting the first round of cocktails, I visualise a cartoon angel on my left shoulder, reminding me of Dr Grant cautioning mental health episodes and alcohol dependency can form part of a vicious circle. Today, I'm in cahoots with the devil on the other side, both of us mesmerised by the barman concocting his brain-cell annihilating potions, adding dashes from numerous bottles at a dizzying rate while the Happy Mondays version of 'Step On' blares.

Our initial rounds comprise general chat. The inevitable bitching about managers. Discussing the football if I'm in John's company. Several cocktails later, I plonk myself beside Shona, a curvy blonde who works in the auditing department, flirting so unsubtly she feels it necessary to keep mentioning her fiancé.

There's a communal decision for a change of scenery so we troop along to The Grosvenor at the West End. The bar is rammed and there's a Cancer Research fundraiser on, with balloons everywhere, and a perky DJ who keeps breaking into Jimmy Savile impressions.

Most of the entourage have stepped down a gear after the cocktail frenzy, switching to lager or shorts. But I'm on Pink Panthers: a snakebite of lager and cider with a blackcurrant dash. Although it tastes like fruit juice, by the time my fourth pint is demolished, the bar is rocking like a train carriage.

My mouth fills with saliva, which always pre-empts a hurling episode. I stumble towards the toilets. As I weave around tables, I tread on a loose balloon. When it bursts I react as if I've blundered into a landmine, leaping from the beer-stained carpet. The whole pub seems to dissolve into mirth. I cough up vomit, splatter my white shirt. Chuckles turn to groans. Nina grabs my sleeve and steers me towards the gents, ordering me to douse myself with water. Robot-like, I comply. Inside, I drench the shirt from a tap until it sticks to me like a foul-smelling skin. Filling the sink, I plunge my head in. When I stagger out, Nina is waiting with my jacket. After I've zipped it to my neck, she propels me towards the door.

The fresh air is welcoming but I feel assailed by the cacophony of traffic and people. We skulk down the lane off Queensferry Street towards the Engine Room. Straightening up for the bouncers, I follow her downstairs. The confines of this cellar bar reverberating with R.E.M., I swerve to the toilets again, hunkering down in the cubicle, face resting in my elbows. I lapse into a stupor. 'Shiny Happy People' fades.

A fist smacks the door. A harsh voice demands to know how much longer I'm going to be. Lurching to my feet, I stagger into the wall, crack my elbow. I blink at my surroundings, no idea how long I've been conked out. Or where. I don't recognise the irate male. Nor can I recall who'll be waiting for me.

Fumbling for the door, I barge past a grey-haired guy, head for the sink. I throw up again. Staring at myself in the mirror I'm shocked by the dishevelled, red-eyed mask that gawks back, gluey saliva trickling from its chin. I exit. After alarming moments when I recognise none of the people scattered around the bar, all of whom are staring, I discover Nina at a corner table.

Tapping her watch, she asks where the fuck I've been. I admit I've been barfing, and my throat's like fucking sandpaper. A pint of lager awaits my attention, as intimidating as a vast plate of stodgy food in some redneck eating contest in the US Bible Belt. After iffy mouthfuls, the drink begins gliding down my throat again. Soothing. I give an exaggerated sigh.

As I'm still recoiling from the effects of peaking so soon, I'm pleased to let her ramble on. Fifteen minutes later, as I'm waiting at the bar, someone taps my shoulder. It's my old buddy, John. We embrace like freed hostages. His brother drummed in First Priority, a new wave band. Ten years before, they had an adjoining practice room to 4 Minute Warning in the former Regent cinema. John often hung around his brother's sessions. Just as Anne and her pals Julie, Lesley and Carol would with us, the girls adding backing vocals to our mad punk cover of 'If I Had a Hammer,' an American folk song made famous by Trini Lopez.

I chatted with John when our paths crossed at the bar or the jukebox in the Regent Buffet, the pub on the corner of Abbeymount where late 1970s youth subcultures – punks, skins, rudeboys, mods, soulboys – guzzled beer and avoided the glares of the older bikers.

We wound up temping beside each other in St Andrew Square in 1987. He's been a regular contact for drinking sessions ever since. I shake hands with the Amazon with her arm wrapped around him and kiss her on the cheek. I've met his current girlfriend before, but to my embarrassment can't recall her name. I always refer to her as Geena. The more I've had to drink, the greater her resemblance to Geena Davis, star of two videos Anne and I have watched, *The Fly* and *Earth Girls Are Easy*. 'Geena' is taller than us both, with cascading brunette hair, wearing a black bodysuit that heightens every sweeping contour of her ample curves. A few years ago she was a Sixth

Year at Portobello High School, a fact that causes his mates no end of childish amusement and *Lolita* gibes.

My cousin Christine's partner, Kenny is a Physics teacher there and remembers her. I muse about the way senior pupils are portrayed in St Trinian's films. While teenagers over the age of consent in uniform might be a perennial fantasy, the reality of succumbing to hormonal urges ruined a colleague's career.

As John orders his next round, I'm thinking of Christine. Ages with Anne, they were thick as thieves as kids, especially during our St Abbs holidays. More like close siblings than cousins, they would spend hours playing together. Ditto her brother Ross and me.

The summer after my discharge from psychiatric care, I used our annual visit to Berwickshire to get wasted on ridiculous chlorpromazine and alcohol cocktails every night. One night after departing a local hostelry, St Veda's, I managed to lose a shoe during a misguided attempt to kick my height. After hopping back to our holiday home, when I collapsed on my bed the room began whirling. Fresh air was the only way to counter the imminent nausea. Deciding to retrace my steps and search for my shoe, I tried rousing Anne and Christine to join my posse. Anne was already snoring. My little cousin insisted my shoe would be so much easier to retrieve in daylight. A voice of reason against my ludicrous notion.

Such madcap behaviour predated my sectioning. Returning from a drunken blowout in Rumours with Grum once, we were skulking along the West Approach Road and an attempt to kick my height led to my slip-on shoe soaring over Fountainbridge Brewery's barbed-wire walls.

Devoid of taxi fares, we often took this route home since it was much quicker than Dundee Street. But this also meant running the risk of being intercepted by police patrols. We were stopped one time and ordered into the back for trespassing in a no-pedestrian zone. Asked our destination, we replied Moat and Shandon. Like the fucking champagne, one of them quipped as we were driven back to Lothian Road. The next time we said Dumbie and were whisked all the way to the Diggers.

I snap out of my reverie when John asks where I've been during my latest binge. My recollections of the earlier portion of the evening are hazy. Alluding to the Billy Connolly skit about Scotsmen in Rome, I admit to having been shouting on Hughey and Ralph. He winks. In the good old days, Splodge would've pulled out the yellow card he fashioned from post-its and waved it at me.

He says Shona and he are off to Madogs if I want to join them. I tell him I'm with a mate from work, will defo pop along after I finish my next beer. I've always been jealous of his confidence compared to my own alcohol-reliant diffidence. Although Shona is a beautiful young woman, I know John can be just as itchy-footed as me where romance is concerned. Maybe the age difference will provide a convenient excuse for him to move on? Having said that, watching them gazing into each other's eyes and whispering small talk, they appear enraptured.

Returning to Nina I grin, suggesting Madogs for the continuation of our pub crawl. But when I gesture in the direction of George Street, my hand sends both our drinks to the floor, alcohol swilling everywhere, glass splintering. Nina shakes her head. She'll be going no further than escorting me to the nearest taxi rank. And it'll be touch and go whether any driver will allow me on board.

46

Hungover Games

The painting dominating the Blue Lagoon's far wall, a kitsch impression of a Pacific paradise, is hidden by the widescreen TV opening onto Hampden Park. It's not even 5 p.m. but the pub is rammed, the bar staff toiling between customers, pumps, gantry, and cash register. As soon as empties are whisked away, fresh pints and chasers replace them in a never-ending relay, against a background din where conversations sound as if they're being conducted by town criers.

My mate Ronnie states he needs a double. His nerves can't cope. The Dons have *got* to nail the fucking Tims. Can't have Septic winning *three* Scottish Cups on the bounce.

I met Ronnie a year ago on one of the buses that pick up at Haymarket, whisking Edinburgh's Old Firm supporters to 'home' games 50 miles away. I grew up supporting a local team but was also drawn to Rangers when I started fuelling my bipolar rollercoaster with lager, cider and vodka, sometimes getting no closer to Ibrox than the Stadium Bar until the time for the return journey.

I was on first-name terms with every barmaid under 40 in that pub, had asked out and been knocked back by all of them. The other week, Cara, a ringer for Ellen Barkin with an hourglass figure and broken nose, surprisingly declined my offer to be whisked off to her city's West End nightspots after her shift. A guy next to me announced I'd had a narrow escape: Cara was a *bead rattler*. I came close to receiving a Glasgow kiss when I retorted only a prick would fixate on beads when fantasising about rattling any of the barstaff.

Ronnie's a dyed-in-the-wool bluenose, complete with a Union Jack tattoo and the predictable repertoire of offensive songs. But extremism aside we get on well, with interests beyond 90 minutes. Like me, he's single. Way more outgoing, although that balance has been tipping the other way in recent months. He sometimes steps into the role of wingman Alex vacated after falling for a striking blonde, Gillian in Buster Brown's. They married on Scottish Cup final day last year.

Although Ronnie wears blue tops on Saturdays - Rangers, Chelsea or Linfield - the prevalence of red or green and white shirts has meant opting for Scotland away. Against the sunlight, its yellow and white hoops are glowing. When he first swaggered through the doors, I was grateful. Since Souness was given a blank chequebook to sign the English internationals denied European football after Heysel, England shirts have started appearing in the Ibrox stands. I admit their latest World Cup anthem by New Order is excellent. But any Scot donning the three lions is football's equivalent of Lord Haw-Haw.

A lot of the Celtic contingent are emphasising the gulf between athletes paid a fortune for sporting the hoops and fans wearing the replicas, anticipating toasting victory, pint after pint. I choked on my Pils at one point. 'Golden Brown' came on the jukebox before the coverage started and I mentioned the Men in Black. Ronnie nodded. *Aye, but check out all the fucking Michelin Men in green.*

Now we're both intent on the TV. The match is still goalless after extra time. The respective squads are gathered around Billy McNeill and Alex Smith. Passing around water bottles. Psyching themselves up for the penalty shootout: the first time the Scottish Cup will have been settled by spot-kicks.

Celtic's Polish defender Dariusz Wdowczyk misses their first attempt to tumultuous applause. When Aberdeen's Brian Grant misses their fourth it becomes deadlocked. At eight-all it goes to sudden death.

My swimming vision notices twin versions of Ronnie. They've thrown their heads back, holding their Buds towards the ceiling. Stoking their nerves.

The camera homes in on Anton Rogan, the Celt's Irish defender. He paces backwards, way beyond the 18-year line. The lens zooms in on a young lad in the east stand, around my age when I was taken to watch Turnbull's Tornadoes. Hands clasped in prayer. Guessing which direction Rogan will strike, Theo Snelders dives to his left, tipping the ball past the post, provoking thunderous acclaim. Aberdeen's number eight, Brian Irvine, paces to the spot. He buries it. Dons fans and their 90-minute sympathisers jump, punching the air, the roaring so intense my ears buzz. Red and white scarves are tossed around. Against the racket, Ronnie shrugs, picking at his bottle's label, muttering about the sheepshaggers being the lesser of two evils. Just.

*

As Ronnie and I stumble into the searing sunshine, past shoppers returning from Princes Street laden with bags, we swig lager from the bottles lifted from a table on the way out, toasting each other. Intimidating, comical, and pathetic. I suggest popping into my parents' house to raid their fridge. This evening they're dining at the Littlejohns, not relatives but close friends of my Grannie. Always Auntie Betty and Uncle Bill to Anne and me growing up.

Before Bill passed away, he and Dad would sometimes drink in the Newmarket Bar by the Chesser slaughterhouse. Bill was older and served in the Gordon Highlanders during World War 2. He was captured at Anzio, spending three years in Stalag IVB in Saxony.

Dad said Bill was a quiet man at the best of times. Never divulged much about his wartime experiences, even when pressed after a few ales. He did mention the Scottish prisoners produced their own newspaper, *The Scotsman*, using quinine stolen from the medical stores to produce the ink. He also described a sub-camp within the camp reserved for Soviet prisoners. Of the tens of thousands who transitted through here, the majority died of typhus. Those that didn't became slaves in Belgian mines. During a rare misty-eyed reminiscence, Bill recalled liberation day in April 1945. Soviet troops entered the camp gates led by an officer riding a white horse.

Tonight they'll listen to Betty, a loquacious Geordie, and her daughter Anne, both Bill's polar opposite, hogging the conversation. Betty making Mum fret as she goes on and on, long tubes of ash accumulating before Anne reminds her to tap them into the ashtray beside her own jackknifed Mores. Dad will attempt to curtail her rambling with a joke he never tires of, suggesting the Queen Mother's blood type is three-parts Gordon's Gin, infuriating the ardent English royalist.

When we get back to the flat, Ronnie and I decide to chill before heading into town for more beers. He dives off to the loo. I decide to phone John and see if he's up for a rendezvous since I missed him last night.

An unknown voice answers, the accent American. He demands rather than asks who's calling. When I tell him it's Mark, John's buddy, the phone magnifies my slurred voice. I giggle. But he remains cagey, his tone like strong coffee against my drunken state. He is confrontational. But it's more than this. I detect he's struggling to remain composed. To suppress fury. Just because I sound as if I've had a few?

I elaborate I bumped into John last night, wondering if he'll be up for a peevo pronto? A lengthy pause. Exasperated breaths. The mysterious American tells me John *isn't available for a peevo fucking pronto*. He wants to know where I last saw John.

I stutter, the Engine Room. I fixate on his strange accent. Trans-Atlantic. Punctuated by Edinburgh glottal stops. I say to him: not being rude, but who's this I'm speaking to?

Jimmy. John's big brother.

The penny drops. I feel a sense of relief. I recall John telling me his brother married an American and emigrated to Chicago. That explains the accent. Not the antagonism. He sounds pissed off about something. Itching to take it out on me. Wondering how to counter his attitude, a story springs to mind.

I could tell him about the time we arrived for practice in the Regent to discover the door to his band's room smashed in. We shifted the remaining amps and an empty guitar case into our room until Shug could phone their guitarist, Donald to explain the situation.

First Priority's equipment was way more high-tech than ours. They'd been going for longer, opening for The Clash at the Glasgow Apollo in January 1980. We supported First Priority in November 1981 when the Regent Buffet's manageress invited both bands to play a benefit gig for Muscular Dystrophy at the Astoria.

I remember that gig for two reasons. One, distancing ourselves from punk, on the verge of changing our name from 4 Minute Warning to Radiate Away, our opening track was an instrumental named 'Trees.' When Ross announced this, someone heckled, *youse've got a song about fucking cheese?* It was also our only gig with a guy called Paul on vocals. Toby's departure led to a succession of auditions, none to our satisfaction. We were always sacking our singers. The Fall in reverse.

As these memories whirl through my mind, I'm also thinking of the way The Clash dissuaded equipment thieves, a common occurrence during the nascent days of the London punk scene. They painted their backline bright pink.

I get as far as mentioning First Priority when he cuts me short. I'm starting to get exasperated. Then he says something that causes the effects of several more of this afternoon's beers to evaporate into the tension of his prolonged silences. Voice cracking, he explains John was attacked. Rushed to St John's Hospital, in Livingston.

It's my turn to be tongue-tied. Shocked, I blurt out, *what happened?* So Jimmy paints the picture. John was in a pub up the town last night with Shona. Madogs. Waiting to get served, he stepped over to the busy bar. Two guys standing there. Arguing. John asked if he could squeeze in. Just trying to buy his girl a drink. One of these cunts, his back to John, not even fucking *looking* at him, lifted his empty glass, fucking *smashed* it into John's face. The doctor said an inch lower would've severed his jugular vein. End of fucking story. He was taken to the intensive care unit at St John's. Due to receive plastic surgery on the deep scarring in his cheek.

Jimmy elaborates he travelled to Scotland with his wife and their baby to introduce his parents to their new grandson, John to his nephew. For all of them to have to deal with *this* crazy shit instead?

After the devastating news, I slam the phone down, bursting into tears. Everything has been put into perspective. Sixty thousand fans baying at 22 men kicking a ball. The inevitable violence that would have terrorised Glaswegian passers-by when Aberdeen's sizeable hooligan crew ran amok.

Ronnie bursts into the room, ordering the kettle on before clocking my maudlin condition. I explain everything. Saturday night is cancelled.

*

It occurs to me how close I came to being there. So much street violence is unprovoked. Random. A lottery. This mindless assault could have happened to anyone who walked into that bar last night.

I recall insisting to Nina I could bluff my way past the Madogs bouncers. I'm a past master at feigning sobriety under the scrutiny of gum-chewing doormen. But she realised I was far too many pints beyond performing such subtle subterfuge.

I stare into the carpet. What twisted motivation could compel someone to launch a glass into a stranger's face? My imagination creates a face for this fucking specimen, like an excerpt from the rogues' gallery on *Crimewatch*. I think of Paul Weller's lyrics about a tube station ambush, of muggers smelling of too many right-wing meetings. Rewind 60 years and the hand that wielded that tumbler in Madogs would be raised in salute towards Mosley.

I prepare a cocktail. Johnny Walker. Gordon's Gin. Lemonade. Select a Laurel and Hardy video. *Way Out West*.

I get to the scene where Stan Laurel, having hidden the deeds to a gold mine about his person, is being assaulted by a femme fatale. Tickling him so hard he is consumed with hysterical laughter. I mimic him until my own ribs are aching. I'll take this video to John's family home over at Boswall when he's fit enough to receive visitors. And the new Inspiral Carpets LP. *Life*. Madchester to take his mind off Madogs. We'll deck ourselves at Stan Laurel and Oliver Hardy, whose entire *raison d'etre* could be summed up in one syllable. Joy.

47

Kidney Bingo

Red Stripes arrayed before me, I delve into the tins, gauging the remaining lager in each by assessing its weight. Gulping some. Draining sips in others. I turn my attention to cans and glasses bunched on neighbouring tables. But my eyelids feel so heavy.

A hand jerks my shoulder. The Queen's Hall logo on this barman's shirt hauls me back to reality. *Wake up or you're out, buddy.*

Extricating myself from the chair, I weave around empty tables towards the bar. The same barman appears. Refuses service and nods at a punter to my left. After starting to pour Guinness that splutters, he informs the lad the barrel needs changed. The moment he's out of sight, another barman appears from a side door. When I request a Red Stripe he eyes me, then passes one over. Handing him a fistful of shrapnel, I lurch in the direction of the pounding rhythm.

I enter the concert hall as a cacophony reaches its breakneck climax. The vocals sound deranged. Something about *freeing my mind and breaking my neck,* the three singers stopping dead at the same moment, the final chord ringing out, dissolving into feedback. Dry ice obscures the shadowy figures on the stage and drifts over the audience cheering 'Underwater Experiences.' Someone keeps bawling: *12XU! 12XU!* I recognise the voice. Toby, one of my mates I arrived with.

I now regret missing so much of Wire's set. Their latest album, *Manscape* was only released two days ago. I was looking forward to hearing their new material. I caught the first few songs, up until one they introduced from the new album, 'Small Black Reptile,' they started with the riff to 'I Am The Fly,' instigating thunderous acclaim. This faded into apprehension.

This is Wire's second-ever foray over the border. The only other Scottish gig they've played was at the Splash Club in Glasgow just before Christmas five years ago. Everyone present knows they never do crowd-pleasers. After losing interest in the dancey bounce-along vibes of the bulk of the *Manscape* songs, I decided to plunder the tins abandoned when roars from the main hall indicated the band's arrival.

As the dry ice dissipates, Colin Newman, Bruce Gilbert, and Graham Lewis are revealed. Robert Gotobed left the band just before this tour started, the remaining trio using the drums and percussion he programmed.

Then I spy Toby. Twinned. Somehow they're on the stage. Next to the Newman doubles. Seizing his microphones. *Give us some hardcore*, they bawl, mouth too close, the growl distorting over the PA.

Two security guys manhandle him past the *Manscape* posters towards the exit. Raising my can, toasting his bravado, the arena starts to spin.

48

Secrets

June 1990

Although I've drunk enough to be seeing double, I try fixing Anne in my sights. *I've got something to tell you.*

Returning from her night out with best friend Lesley, my sister surveys the empty red wine bottles. Chased with Diamond Whites. I'm on the last tin of 8.2% cider from a six-pack so her expression reveals her dilemma. Is this just the drink talking? Again. Something weightier? She tells me she's all ears.

I need to get this off my chest. I've never told anyone before. Not even Mum and Dad. *Especially* not them. Wish I had at the time, though. Not now.

What is it, Mark? You're scaring me.

Fortify myself with a slug of Diamond White. Okay. When I was 13, I was invited to a church outing. A Sunday school picnic. By a pal from my class. Andy. He went to Cairns

Memorial church. So. At this picnic, there was a guy. Don't know if he was a Sunday school teacher. Or just one of the congregation. Anyway. Let me tell you about this *cunt*.

Anne purses her lips.

He asked me to chum him to fill urns, you know? For tea. He took me into this outhouse. And.

Another gulp.

Then he fucking... sexually assaulted me.

Oh my *God*, Mark. What... What did he do to you?

He toyed with me. Groped me. He never got his fucking cock out or anything. But he felt me up for a while. Maybe only five, ten minutes. But it seemed longer. Time stood still. Well. I was in shock. But what made it worse... He reminded me of Ian Brady. Photos of that horrible, horrible cunt. I was in shock. I honestly thought he might strangle me.

Couldn't you have told the adults that were there? Cairns Memorial? That was the school minister's church, wasn't it?

Aye. Reverend MacDonald. His wife was our English teacher in third year. No. Like I said. I was in shock. Dumb-struck. Part of me stayed in shock for years.

Anne stands up. Embraces me. Are you going to tell the folks?

No. No way. I've kept my secret from them long enough. I don't want that image inside their heads. Especially Mum. Her wee boy in the hands of that fucking predator.

I shrug. Now there are three people who know the truth about what happened one day in 1976.

Wow. I don't know what to say, Mark. That's horrible. The fucking pervert. D'you think he still goes to that church?

He may well do. Experts at covering their tracks, these creeps. And kids are easily terrified into silence. I was so shy, anyway. A devilishly handsome young boy...

Anne manages a smile.

... quiet as a church mouse. He must've thought he'd hit the nonce jackpot.

49

Protest And Survive

Hearing Anne's bedroom door closing, I finish the cider. Check the time. Just gone one. Seven hours of drunken stupor then up for overtime. Dropping the can into the bucket, I spy yesterday's *Evening News*. A lightbulb moment. Rummaging in drawers, I search for paper. Scissors. Pritt Stick.

*

I poke the glue pen into the 'Y' to complete the message. Holding the flyer aloft, I beam at my artwork, its collision of font styles and sizes reminiscent of punk artwork. Aping a communication from a kidnapper. **FuCK WALLACE MERCENARY**

Earlier this week, Wallace Mercer, Heart of Midlothian FC's chairman, announced his intention to 'merge' his own club with Hibernian FC to form a superclub. This 'Edinburgh United' might even still play in maroon with the same badge over their hearts. Based at Tynecastle. Or some new stadium to be built on protected land owned by his friend David Murray.

The extinction of Hibs, a 115-year-old club dear to my own heart, will be collateral damage. This has triggered something in me. I've been obsessing about this, not *just* this, but *especially* this, over the past few days.

I've only been Anne's lodger since April. But feel everything happening at once. Moving away from home. The new job. The 'Hands Off Hibs' campaign. Nightcaps. Not usually including wine *and* cider concoctions on school nights. But a bottle of red opened every other evening.

Alcohol has always proved an effective if short-term lubricant in countering the innate shyness dealt such an incapacitating blow in 1976. At a time when a reasonable percentage of youngsters begin developing confidence and socialising skills, spurred on by approaching adulthood and the blossoming of sexuality, I often fixated on the horror of those moments in that pervert's clutches.

I struggled, making few friends at secondary compared to my boisterous posse of mates from Craiglockhart: Ian, Barry, Crowie, Sparky, Clarkey, Stevie, Donald. It happened during the summer holidays. When I moved onto Third Year I tended to retreat into my bedroom after school, where I would complete my homework with minimal effort, then spend the rest of my leisure time seeking escapism.

I found the best way to forget about real trauma was to bury my nose in fantasy novels – Isaac Asimov, J R R Tolkein, Robert Heinlein, John Wyndham, John Norman – hard or progressive rock blaring inside my headphones. Black Sabbath. Blue Oyster Cult. Uriah Heep. Status Quo. Queen. And Kiss. I was big on Kiss, Gene Simmons dominating my poster display in all his lurid make-up and fake blood drooling glory.

When I did venture out of my room, I'd be glued to the TV, to *The Sweeney*, *The Water Margin*, or comedies like *The Benny Hill Show* or *It Ain't Half Hot Mum*. Unfettered by political correctness or indeed, for the most part, comedy.

I might well have retreated further into an insular, hermit-like and virginal existence if it wasn't for timing. Around a year or so on from that sexual assault, an inflammatory new music scene began emerging. When the media latched onto this sub-culture it was dubbed punk rock.

The memories spark a frenetic excitement. Heading into my bedroom, I don my headphones, bowing to my collection. I didn't just listen to this frenzied rock 'n' roll in the same way I enjoyed playing my Queen or Led Zeppelin or Black Sabbath albums. I developed an insatiable desire for the exhilarating and profane singles these innovative bands were releasing: three-minute outbursts of energy distilled into vinyl, packaged in lurid sleeves also perfect for bedroom wall decor.

I select *Damned Damned Damned*, popping side 2 onto my record player. Lifting the needle to the final four tracks, I ease up the volume... *one two three go... See Her Tonite... 1 of the 2... one two three, oh she's so... Messed Up... Hey Keith... Feel Alright*, the swaggering tribute to Iggy Pop and The Stooges. *Outa mind on a Saturday night...*

The Damned. The Clash. The Jam. The Sex Pistols. Wire. Buzzcocks. The Saints. Adam and the Ants. Subway Sect. The Fall. Siouxsie and the Banshees. The Stranglers. And so many more. They transcended labels as prosaic as pop or rock. Seizing the zeitgeist, like a surfer, this became the soundtrack to your life.

Key for me, the combination of stripped-back riffs and acerbic lyrics wasn't just a metaphoric two-finger salute to the establishment, it was the voice of disaffected youth. And who could be more disaffected than a bright but shy Edinburgh teenager whose memories of falling victim to a nonce were still so recent?

Punk sparked a fuse that became a conflagration. Encompassing art. Literature. Language. Fashion. Politics. Attitudes. Inclusivity. Female musicians took centre stage like never before. Performers found a voice to counter homophobia. Wayne County and the Electric Chairs courted controversy, not just for their unpredictable performances and their single, '(If You Don't Wanna Fuck Me Baby) Fuck Off!!' featuring a teenage Jools Holland's first studio session. Also for Wayne becoming Jayne, the first openly transgender rock star.

Next up, Visitors. 'Electric Heat.' A perfect meld of rawer punk and futuristic electronica. Before post-punk, they were punkier. The Deleted. Famously supporting Scars at the 1978 Anti-Nazi League Carnival at Craigmillar Festival. Rock Against Racism prompted youths from every ethnic or social background to come together and celebrate common passions. Fans were galvanized to do so much more than just attend concerts – in the case of The Slits or Eater, performed by kids your own age. Punk was proactive.

Mark Perry of Alternative TV and journalist Danny Baker wrote a fanzine called *Sniffin' Glue* that not only chronicled the bands and reinforced the scene's defining DIY ethic, they encouraged fans to create their own fanzines. Another zine, *Sideburn*, printed an illustration of three chords, captioned: "This is a chord, this is another, this is a third. Now form a band."

This prompts my next choice. Alternative TV's 'Life,' Mark Perry seething in irony, listing life's lowpoints. *Growing old. Tramps lying dead in the road.*

To the amazement of Deep Purple adoring mates, neighbours, and schoolteachers, I embraced punk. Those of the latter who hadn't been party to this inconsequential blip on their radar got the message at a school disco when I launched myself from my seat when the DJ played 'No More Heroes.' Enflamed by vodka and blackcurrant, I leapt around and bounced up and down on my own for three minutes 25 seconds, while most onlookers gawked as if I had streaked onto the dancefloor.

Guys I knew from Tynecastle High reacted to that fanzine advice and started their own band, The Accidents. Their anarchic early performances became a focal point.

My next choice. The original of a song they covered. Neon Hearts. 'Regulations.'

When you weren't going to watch local groups or attending gigs at Clouds, the Astoria, the Nite Club above the Playhouse, or at Edinburgh or Heriot-Watt University student unions where you had to coax students into signing you in, you made weekend pilgrimages to Edinburgh's numerous record shops. Buying the latest singles. Fanzines. Badges. T-shirts. Posters.

You chatted with kindred spirits outside Bruce's on Rose Street. The Other Record Shop on the High Street. Ripping Records on the Bridges. You bought stuff, swapped stuff, and if you didn't have enough to purchase a cherished item you might resort to shoplifting stuff.

You sometimes took the train through to Glasgow where there were even more record shops crammed into a small radius, or head to the Apollo – for The Damned, Sham 69, The Stranglers – then leg it back to Queen Street station for the last train to Haymarket. Skulking into doorways when you spotted prowling Teddy Boys.

Reminding myself of the time we saw Sham 69 in Glasgow and they were joined by Steve Jones and Paul Cook for their encore, I drop the needle. Jimmy Pursey's manic laughter. 'Borstal Breakout.'

You hung around in youth clubs – Merchiston Boy's Club, Cephas Cellar, the Chesser, the Telecomms Club – where you could take along your own singles to pogo to. You got into skirmishes with Northern Soulboys or, latterly, Mods. In the gloom, on rickety chairs, your breath reeking of Tennent's lager and vodka slugged from a communal bottle while pinching your nose, you snogged punkettes, twirling your tongue around the moist taste of Embassy Regal.

No one else knew my reasons for gravitating to a subculture the tabloids equated with the erosion of Western civilisation. But punk was a defence mechanism. A shell to skulk behind. The paradox was this shell was gaudy, attracting undue attention spanning a gamut of reactions, from ridicule to outright violence.

Asking Mum to sew zips into flared school trousers or Anne to knit a string vest like Paul Simenon's was akin to the behaviour of those self-conscious individuals drawn to becoming actors.

The world is full of performers, on stage or behind microphones, who relish inhabiting the persona of an alter-ego, only to retreat into their coy selves in the sanctuary of their dressing rooms. An archetypical example would have to be David Bowie. Off-stage, self-effacing, almost shy but charming. On-stage or in the studio, the ever-morphing chameleon and obsessive artist.

A shrinking violet myself, I thought nothing of dressing the part. At a time when I should've been considering a 6th Year at Tynecastle after failing to secure decent Higher grades for university, I ditched school. In the summer of 1979, you could claim the dole straight away. At one point I was covering my mate Barry's paper round while signing on at the Broo next to Goldbergs at Tollcross. After cashing my first giro at the Shandon Post Office on the Friday, I took a 35 bus to the High Street, popped into Phoenix Record Shop, and splashed out on *Scared to Dance* by The Skids, Wire's new single, 'A

Question of Degree,' and the recent Joy Division album, *Unknown Pleasures*.

Now I select Joy Division's 'Transmission,' flipping onto the b-side. 'Novelty.' A gem.

After a summer of vinyl and long lies, my Uncle Alex, the Glasgow branch manager for Scottish Widows, spoke to a colleague in the Edinburgh head office in Dalkeith Road, and I was offered a post without even attending an interview. I endured three years and 10 months of calculator tapping and form-filling, working out insurance policy quotations in the antiquated pre-PC environment.

Where 90% of my colleagues conformed to the shirt, tie and suit stereotype, I showed up in tousled hair, Crisis and Poison Girls badges pinned to my Harrington, drainpipe trousers, and lumbering thick crepe soles that earned me the nickname 'Frankenstein.'

What next? Poison Girls. 'Persons Unknown.' Takes me back to the Astoria, 10 years ago. They supported Crass. I took Anne. I was 17, my sister 15. The first support act was a spoken word performer, Annie Anxiety. Skinheads and mohicans clustered at the front. Covered her in a blizzard of spit. Continued gobbing on the Crass and Poison Girls' stage backdrops. Afterwards, the so-called 'Livvi Skins' rampaged up and down Abbeyhill, assaulting punks. Only one of Steve Ignorant's mantras of 'Anarchy, Peace and Freedom,' had been taken to heart. No wonder Paul Weller felt compelled to decry punk's bloodletting tribalism and Doctor Marten's apocalypse in 'A Bomb in Wardour Street.'

From 1978 I was listening to what constituted 'post-punk' with Barry. In my class throughout primary, our paths diverged after he passed the entrance exam for George Watson's, the local fee-paying secondary, and I failed. But we kept in touch at Scouts, the Youth Fellowship – Sunday School for older teenagers – and our love of XTC, Wire, The Stranglers, Magazine, and Ultravox. *Pink Flag*, *White Music*, and *The Scream* were particular obsessions.

Despite his current tastes, he still had a Yes poster appended to his bedroom wall, *Tales From Topographic Oceans*, and once described a Genesis concert in terms of Peter Gabriel's costumes, the band's musicianship when they launched into elaborate solos, the light show, the glossy programme. Seeing The Mekons at Clouds or hearing The Clash on John Peel's Radio 1 shows made me want to rush out and buy a guitar. I did so when I got my first pay Scottish Widows cheque: a Gibson copy.

My next choice is the 12" single Barry eventually sold me after industrial-level badgering. The white vinyl edition of Ultravox's 'Quiet Men.' Then I delve further into their past, replacing guitarist Robin Simon with Stevie Shears. 'Young Savage,' the one Toby and I would freak out to at the Merky.

I was a member of their fan club. Upon joining, they sent me the A2-sized posters of *Ha!-Ha!-Ha!* and *Systems of Romance* still holding pride of place opposite my bed. When Midge Ure became Foxx's replacement, the fan club sent a letter requesting I begin paying a subscription. I declined.

The post-punk scene in central Scotland was such fertile ground. In Edinburgh, a cathartic moment was The Clash rocking up to the Playhouse on Saturday 7th May 1977 for the fourth gig of their White Riot Tour, one month on from releasing their debut album, and with their new drummer, Topper Headon. Support came from The Jam, Buzzcocks, The Slits, and Subway Sect. Audience members that night went on to form The Dirty Reds, evolving into The Fire Engines, Orange Juice, The Flowers, Josef K, Boots for Dancing, The Rezillos, and the local band we all took to our hearts: Scars.

I'm compelled to play 'Adult/ery,' an adrenaline-rush of a debut single from the band once described by Mark E Smith as his favourite because they were The Fall's polar opposite. Followed by the spine-tingling 'Horrorshow,' infectious riffing by Edinburgh's answer to Mick Ronson, Paul Research, while Bobby King's cuts and pastes elements of Anthony Burgess's 'A Clockwork Orange,' giving a delirious wanton voice to the bowler hat wearing *droogs*.

Legend has it that trailblazing concert also spawned Scotland's renowned DIY record labels: Bob Last forming Fast Product in the capital, whose first releases included Northern English bands The Mekons, Human League, Gang of Four, that Scars 45, Adult/ery; and at the west end of the M8, Alan Horne initiating Postcard Records.

My first band was formed at the tail end of punk's first wave, coinciding with The Damned reforming, Captain Sensible replacing Brian James on guitar and releasing 'Love Song.' Mates from Stenhouse, Shandon, Gorgie; Pauline and Raymond, an item, and Toby, from my year at Tynecastle, became vocalist, drummer and bassist.

Falling into that rarer but ultra-cool category of having a female frontperson, like the Banshees, X-Ray Spex and Penetration, we thought up an appropriate name. The Seduced. We invested in gear. Toby, who'd left school by then and was an apprentice car mechanic, splashed out on a beautiful Fender like J J Burnel's.

Raymond, a defector from the Northern Soul camp who'd been an enthusiast of coach trips to Wigan and Blackpool all-nighters within the past few months, started kneading egg whites into his wedge hairstyle to create the requisite spikes. Bought a drumkit which he spraypainted. Pauline, the younger sister of The Accidents' drummer, had access to mikes.

I mustered a few three-chord riffs and a passable rendition of 'Art-I-Ficial' by X-Ray Spex. We progressed to daubing the band name in lurid lettering on the launderette on the corner of Ashley Terrace before the initial enthusiastic spark floundered with Pauline and Raymond's on/off teenage romance.

X-Ray Spex up next, the B-side of 'Identity,' 'Let's Submerge.' This leads onto the even more ferocious flip side, 'I Am a Cliché.'

I followed The Axidents (as they tweaked their name) to every gig, from their debut at the Gorgie War Memorial to the YMCA in South St Andrew Street supporting The Exploited, Kilburnie to Forfar's Reid Hall. At the latter event, they were supported by Burning Flags, Twisted Nerve, and the Sceptix. The quartet shared bills under the moniker, 'Capital Chaos.'

Hordes of locals gatecrashed and proceeded to pick fights with teenage punks. This degenerated into a full-blown riot. The bands and their fans beat a hasty tactical retreat onto the stage. Hoisted the massive curtains shut to block the hail of pint glasses.

Tayside punk-bashers kept clambering onto the stage like pirates boarding a stricken ship, to be beaten back by mike stands. Shug's cymbals were deployed like martial arts weapons. During the melee, one infiltrator leapt through the curtains, was shoved overboard, hauling me with him. I saw biker jackets. Curling into a ball, feet lashed from the gloom. Big boots. Regulars from The Stag round the corner? AC/DC fans? As blows rained in, I imagined tumbling into a cauldron of Altamont Hell's Angels. Eventually, I scrambled back onto the stage. The Forfar cops were slow to react. Every window in the coach was smashed. 'Capital Chaos' indeed.

The Axidents recorded a brilliant demo. John Peel played a track from it. But they didn't get to play that night and the violent scenes prompted The Axidents' gifted new guitarist, Derek, to leave. He joined The Associates on keyboards.

I bumped into Shug and bassist Ross on their way to a CND meeting in Shandon. They invited me to join the new venture they were excited about, a post-punk band they intended as a vehicle for anti-nuclear warfare politics.

In true punk style, there were no songs yet, but they already had the name, which Ross had embossed on stickers at the paper merchants warehouse where he worked. 4 Minute

Warning. Those stickers became a familiar decoration on LRT buses, clustering around the upstairs seating, at the back.

Barely progressing beyond those three chords mentioned in *Sideburn*, I had big creepers to fill. Derek's mastery of his Gibson Les Paul was reminiscent of Steve Jones, Johnny Thunders or Derwood from Generation X. But I agreed, glowing with excitement.

4 Minute Warning became a key part of my teenage life. Ross and Shuggy had developed into skilled musicians. Toby had given up on playing bass but he was the only choice for our singer. Confident and charismatic, he could hold a tune – his Hogmanay party pieces centred on note-perfect renditions of Frank Sinatra and Dean Martin rather than anything as cliched as rehashing Joe Strummer.

As well as experimenting with rock riffs, interspersed with reggae and even proto-funk, I loved writing lyrics. For someone saddled by introversion, here was the ultimate form of self-expression.

Crouching to the records, I pick out my next choice, the Red Beat 12" EP, 'Machines in Motion,' released on Malicious Damage, Killing Joke's label. With its apocalyptic cover featuring soldiers in gas masks against a mushroom cloud nuclear denotation, this was also staple listening for my band. Amazingly, an early incarnation of Red Beat featured three brothers of synth-pop *Top Of The Pops* regular Howard Jones.

Looking back on my 4 Minute Warning writing, it was rudimentary, time-stamped as 1980. This was the height of the Cold War menace, with the UK Government producing leaflets entitled 'Protect and Survive' that outlined how the continuing arms race and the concept of 'mutually assured destruction' relied on the population accepting the hypothetical possibility of nuclear war.

You were encouraged to learn how to survive this Armageddon. The leaflet suggested painting your windows white and fashioning a shelter by unscrewing a door to wedge against a wall, assuring you that cowering beneath six inches of wood would deflect the blast from a 475-kiloton nuclear detonation. That it was common knowledge there were underground fallout shelters for members of the establishment in the event of the actual four-minute warning sounding was the ultimate expression of Britain's class structure, of a society segregated into haves and have-nots. Those worthy of living and those not.

4 Minute Warning may have been a line from the first single by Killing Joke, our favourite post-punk band and biggest inspiration, but it was also the red line of our politics. Shug daubed his drumkit with the CND logo and their alternative slogan: 'Protest and Survive,' the antithesis of Protect and Survive's horrifying, dehumanising propaganda. A few copies of my original lyric sheets have survived, in a meticulous teenage script.

The graffitied pages I've produced today remind me of the punk fanzines we once cobbled together in 4 Minute Warning: teenage angst distilled into typewriter text, the headings cut from newspapers and pieced together like blackmail notes, the mock-ups mass-produced on Xerox machines. Dad used to do some of them for me in his own office, after hours. I transcribed the words to one of our songs, left copies in Bruces, Hot Wax, and The Other Record Shop. Somehow this made its way into an early edition of *I.D. Magazine*. But instead of frothing about copyright infringement, I basked in the kudos of mass readership.

By the 1980s punk had moved way beyond constricting dress codes and three-chord templates. 'Did You Know Wrong' led to *Metal Box*. '12XU' to *154*. Warsaw to 'Blue Monday.' 'White Riot' to *Sandinista!* and its wondrous collision of reggae, funk, jazz, dub, calypso, disco and rap. It had also mutated into 'Oi,' epitomised by studded leather jackets and furious delivery. Heavy metal on speed, with shoulder-length hair replaced by mohicans or skinheads.

4 Minute Warning changed our name twice, from Radiate Away to Desperation A.M. Like so many bands at that time, our image also altered, chameleon-like, although I was last to relinquish those thick-soled Teddy Boy-parody shoes once so *de rigueur* for everyone from Johnny Rotten to Killing Joke, colluding with the rest of the guys in adopting colourful shirts, baggy trousers, and pointed boots. Interviewed for a fanzine, we claimed stylistic alongside musical influences, now citing Bauhaus and Duran Duran.

Poking into the 'B' segment of the alphabetic sequence, I find 'Bela Lugosi's Dead,' the former's Gothic dub masterpiece.

Toby fell for a local girl, Laura, one of the Abbeyhill teenagers who used to drift into our rehearsals, leaving to focus on the fatherhood that followed. Desperation A.M. were joined by a new singer, Looby, a mate of the band who shared our practice room, a bunch of Ayr ex-pats called Little Big Dig.

A hometown mate of his, Coddy became our lead guitarist. I was relegated to rhythm guitar, and although a new dimension was added to our sound, my demotion extinguished my enthusiasm. Desperation A.M. split.

I was invited to play bass, then guitar, for Little Big Dig, led by Tom, another Ayr mate of Looby and Coddy. After a two-year relationship, me and Louise, a lovely punkette hairdresser, split. A void opened in my life which I filled with the new band and binge drinking. I become a regular clubber, in those days, Valentino's, JJ's, Outer Limits, Mad Hatter's.

'Bela Lugosi's Dead' was their debut single, but it lasts nine minutes and 38 seconds. Daniel Ash's sweeping, reverb-heavy, echoey guitar slices are hypnotic. My eyelids are getting heavy. I think of reviving my aural senses by shoving on Punishment of Luxury's 'Brain Bomb.' But fatigue is enveloping me.

So much for the cultural cyclones swirling around my past. Tomorrow, I know I'll feel an even more acute sense of needing to grasp at things to do in my life. To express myself in direct ways.

I think of the flyers. Mercer's dream of untold riches at the cost of killing Hibernian is yet another iron thrust into the bipolar foundry.

The other day I was browsing some article in one of the Sundays when I was visiting my folks: 'Ways the impact of childhood emotional abuse can be revealed in adulthood.'

Although I was skimming this while guzzling pre-dinner sherries, a few points stuck.

'You prefer to be surrounded by toxicity.'

'You criticise yourself for the smallest mistakes but accept others' bad behaviour.'

'You have low self-worth and settle for less than you deserve.'

'You dismiss compassion and kindness because it feels uncomfortable.'

That final one was a metaphoric ice pick to the head. Of all the aspects of that nightmarish afternoon at the picnic, one of the worst was the way it crippled me emotionally. As a family, we have always been tactile, tender in expressing our unconditional love. Mum would wrap an arm around me. Dad might ruffle my hair. A little more awkwardly, Anne and I would embrace on birthdays, on Christmas Day. In the aftermath of the sexual assault, the moment I felt anyone touching me, I would flinch and transform to stone. How I despised that fucking creep for forging such terrible circumspection.

But for the moment, I just want to focus on losing myself to dreams.

50

1875 - 1990

Scuffing into the office at the back of 10, I aim for my chair. Nearly miss.

Alison shakes her head. Marko... Showing up for work late. Stinking like a brewery. And what's in the bag? You brought a carryout and all?

Wish I *had* brought a few tinnies, Al. Could do with the hair of the dog.

Flicking on my PC, I log in, then turn to her again. Just something I need to do before I get started. Winking, I lift the carrier bag.

Last night's wine and cider lingers. Placing a palm against the corridor wall to steady myself, I barge into the photocopy room. Tip the bag's contents onto a table. A4 sheets. Rangers scarf. Madchester bucket hat. Opening the stationery cupboard, I delve into a box containing rolls of white file stickers.

Selecting a green marker pen, I write *HANDS OFF HIBS* onto 30 labels. Festoon the scarf and hat.

Most kids choose the team their parents, step-parents, older siblings or mates follow. Brought up in Shandon and attending Craiglockhart primary, a feeder school for Tynecastle High, most of my pals chose locally. Heart of Midlothian. Dad had no interest in football. But he was Irish. I chose Hibernian.

It took a season or two of intermittent cajoling to wear him down. Finally relenting, he took me to my first match at Easter Road when I was 11. For most fans, once that course has been set it can never be altered. But my own trajectory hit that buffer in 1976. The dismal encounter at Carberry Tower affected me in so many ways. One major outcome was a complete dousing of my enthusiasm for the football, imposing a twisted outlook.

Graeme, a new pal after moving into third year later that summer, wore a Rangers scarf to school, plastered in badges bearing the 'red hand of Ulster.' After telling him my dad was an Ulsterman, he said that if he was a 'proddy,' surely he was a Gers man, too? I replied he preferred visits to the dentist than taking me to Easter Road. That he was from Monaghan, an atheist, and favoured Irish reunification meant the pencil's lead was snapped long before any 'proddy' box would ever be ticked.

But Graeme also described escapades when travelling on the Jardine supporters' bus with his big brother every Saturday. This reminded me of my cousins from Whitley Bay, Jimmy and David, Newcastle United supporters, describing Rangers fans rampaging across St James Park during an Inter-City Fairs Cup tie in May 1969, and how the same blue army 'took' Manchester United's Stretford End during a 'friendly' in March 1974.

I bought Iggy Pop's new album, *Brick by Brick* last weekend. In the longest track, 'Neon Forest,' he sings about Americans taking drugs as a form of psychic defence. Maybe that was the reason for such ambiguous allegiances back then. The warped notion that Rangers colours, telegraphing the apex predators of 1970s British hooligan subculture, would have deterred that pervert. My psychic defence.

Eventually swamped by even more mercurial teenage passions – punk and post-punk – my interest in football declined again. A couple of years later, a Scottish Widows workmate, Alan, a bluenose, invited me to a match. For the next few seasons, again with enthusiasm ebbing and flowing, I tagged along to the odd game. I still looked out for Hibs results. Celebrated the rare occasions we won Edinburgh derbies. Then Alan got engaged. Gave up on the football. But his wee brother, Ross remained part of our drinking crew, and he was a Hibee. His more conventional Easter Road loyalties were an excuse to duet 'Glory Glory to the Hibees' as we weaved from Madogs to Buster's every weekend.

After receiving my Publishing diploma from Napier, I applied for job after job, eventually drifting into the open-ended temp work. The monthly pay cheques made the lengthy hours of compulsory overtime worthwhile. But the longer this lasted, the less I could see beyond this dangling carrot other than a void. My moods would swing from the highs of weekend binges to the week day lows, the football just another transient escape.

Fixating on alternative guitar music, especially The Fall, The Smiths, Echo and The Bunnymen, and Bhundu Boys, I could take or leave my odd two-tiered loyalties. Trio, actually, as I also added Meadowbank Thistle to the puzzling cocktail.

I went to Meadowbank matches with my good mate, Brian who drew perplexed glances with the yellow and black scarf he used to wear to Tynecastle. Brian was the writing partner on my first foray into fiction. We contributed alternate hand-written chapters to a space opera epic emulating the *Star Wars* trilogy, injected with elements of our other passions, *Space 1999* and Asimov's *Foundation*. Also big on Jeff Wayne's *War of the Worlds* and ELO, he would castigate my Killing Joke badges and creepers.

When I experienced my first breakdown, the initial diagnosis was 'paranoid schizophrenic episode,' later revised to bipolar, although a Venn diagram would show these ellipses overlapping in many areas. On the sleeve of The Fall single 'Kicker Conspiracy,' Mark E Smith refers to 'the strip of schizophreens.' Much of his lyric writing is cryptic, but I interpreted that as the ambiguity of team colours. Not for the majority of supporters. But the star players kissing the crests of whichever club happened to be paying their exorbitant salaries at that time. The glory hunters switching allegiances based on the contents of trophy cabinets. And the chemically imbalanced. My eccentric three-tiered devotion's greatest dichotomy: Hibs

v. Rangers and being surrounded by weegie accents baying at the *AIDS-carrying bastards*.

Recuperating from the total breakdown in 1987 there was that 'eureka moment' during art therapy when I began emerging from my psychosis by painting a football top. Not royal blue. Green. Like that Cat Stevens song, memorably covered by Rod Stewart, 'The First Cut is the Deepest,' this sentiment could apply to any of your first loves.

This season I've been to Ibrox many times, give or take those occasions I've drunk so many snakebites in the Stadium Bar I've zoned out in a corner and never made it to any turnstile, waking one time to discover my pockets rifled and wallet gone. But nothing, no level of bipolar mania or excess alcohol will match the way my childhood heart would swell with pride when Turnbull's Tornadoes took the field.

A prime example of my atypical allegiances would be the *Evening News* poster celebrating Hibernian's Scottish League Cup win in 1972. This souvenir once held pride of place on my bedroom wall and accompanied me when I left home. The moment news broke of Wallace Mercer's audacious scheme to exterminate the club, this creased memento, with its centremost illustration of Jimmy O'Rourke's winning diving header bulleting past Evan Williams, was Blue Tacked back into pole position. Next to it, a clipping from the *Shoot* magazine my cousin John brought to the Ward 5 visiting room: goalscorers Robert Fleck, Davie Cooper and Iain Durrant cradling this silverware 15 years and multiple traumas later.

Although Hibernian's Irish roots are downplayed compared to the equivalent sentiments where Glasgow Celtic are concerned, I've always been proud to be half-Scottish, half-Irish. Dad was born in 1921 in what had only just been christened the Irish Free State. Mum came from Craigentinny, a few bus stops from Easter Road, big brother Alex a devotee of the Famous Five.

Working for Reid Employment after college, a good drinking buddy was Keith, a Hibs Boy. But I'd also got to know Graeme's buddies from what had been renamed the Union Jack bus. Some of the younger lads defected to the Hibs crew. Many of the scarfers were not averse to alcohol-soaked violence. There has always been a chink of paranoia about falling victim to sexual assault again, even if this threat has receded the further I've grown from childhood. No matter how remote, this mishmash of allies somehow made this possibility diminish. Falling victim to a pervert did many things to my mind as my teens unfolded, not least introducing this weird Jekyll and Hyde dynamic to my football allegiances.

Your first football match is a special moment in anyone's life. Dad taking me to a January 1974 Scottish Cup tie against Kilmarnock, which we won 5-2, with goals by Alex Edwards, Pat Stanton, John Blackley, and two by Jimmy O'Rourke, was an electrifying experience. Stanton on the scoresheet! Club captain, three times Scotland captain, and great-great-nephew of one of Hibernian's founders and first captain, Michael Whelahan.

Back in the present again. I stare at the trays stacked with 100 copies of flyers. Collating these sheets, I feed the second master copy onto the photocopier. This is even more incendiary.

*

Alison's not at her desk. There are only two of us in; she's singing The Soup Dragons while stirring coffee in the wee kitchen. Placing the flyers into neat stacks around my PC, I go onto all fours. Crawling over to her desk, I wheel her chair aside, then skulk underneath. Stifling giggles, I pull the chair closer. She returns, crooning about being free to get her booze. Any old time.

There's your coffee, unless you're kipping in the store cupboard, you headbanger, she murmurs. I bite my lip. *What's all this?* She's flipping through the sheets. Wallet... *Mercenary... The fuck?*

The moment she tugs her chair out the way, I seize her flared jeans. She shrieks. Wriggling from my hiding place, I'm consumed with laughter. Her face is florid and her coffee has sprayed the striplights.

Marko, you idiot!

She takes in the scarf I've draped around my neck. The bucket hat.

You're a maddo. I mean. *What the actual fuck?* You can get a cloth. My coffee went all over the shop. Plus. What's with all these mental photocopies? Weirdest Scottish Office correspondence I've ever seen. And what's with the get-up? You off to a fancy dress party? What's the theme? One Flew Over the Cuckoo's Nest?

In the immortal words of John Foxx. Ha. Ha. Ha.

John who?

Never mind. I'm not off to a party, Al. I'm going to be handing these out at the Hands Off Hibs rally. And Leith pubs. I'm trying to save my football club.

Which one? Hibs stickers? A Rangers scarf? You're off your head.

Where would I start to explain? The explanations whirring inside my head all seem meaningful to me. I also appreciate, *only* me.

I'm trying to finish my work so I can get the 12.10 train back to Dunfie. You better clean up the mess.

Shite. There's coffee all over the flyers.

Whose fault's that?

Lifting those nearest the top, I scrunch them and ball them into my bin. Then I drape a dry page over her keyboard.

Reaching for the cigarette tucked behind my ear, I spark it. During overtime we're permitted to smoke at our desks, a concession Alison, having taken advantage of the office's corporate membership for Marco's Leisure Centre, detests.

Add insult to injury, why don't you, Marko? She waves her hands. Glancing at this sheet, she shakes her head, shoves it back onto my desk. Her PC becomes the focus of her attention.

My mate Martin writes for the Rangers fanzine, *Follow Follow*. He asked me to write an article about today's rally, containing quotes from Hibees and honorary Hibees attending. I've already got my first one, a simple poem written by my line manager, Brian Connolly. If the first person I ever cheered myself hoarse for scoring was Alex Edwards in the early 1970s, his was Joe Baker in the late 1950s.

Mercy, Mr Mercer. Do you want to kill our dreams? The true heart of Hibernian. Will always beat in green.

I take a lingering draw. Alison wafts at the smoke. When I started here I'm sure I came across as a decent, quiet lad, perhaps prone to many beers during Friday afternoon drinking sprees. But diffident. A few weeks later my mind seems to be in ever-increasing turmoil.

Hibernian today are as Scottish as Edinburgh but named after the Emerald Isle, formed as a charity to help destitute immigrants in the Cowgate of the 1870s. So many have crossed the Irish Sea in search of a better life to be met with derision. Discrimination. Violence. Demeaning nicknames. Dad bought his one-way ferry ticket in the 1940s, although getting a job in GPO supplies in London was nowhere near fleeing poverty, pogroms or famine.

My cigarette is almost down to the filter when I suck another draw. I glance at the papers strewn over my desk, consider the quota of forms I was supposed to have processed by now. I've done three out of the 25 expected this morning.

Instead, I begin rambling to Alison about men in suits who regard communities as irrelevant compared to squeezing moolah from tens of thousands of punters every week.

Al. If Mercer gets what he wants, Hibs will become another footnote in the history of Scottish football. Mentioned the same way older Glaswegians reminisce about Third Lanark. The Thirds won the Scottish Cup more recently than Hibs but were liquidated in 1967 while forty K in the red. *Ironic*. Their colours were red.

Frustrated at the lack of response I glare at her. Scowling, she tugs earphones from where they were nestling in her long tresses. Harsh techno blares.

51

A Matter Of Life And Death

I bunch fistfuls of flyers into my jean pockets, dump surplus piles into a paper bin. Exiting the office, I sprint to Shandwick Place and jump on a bus to London Road. The 26 passes the canopy stretching above the Ross Bandstand on Princes Street Gardens. Someone has shinned up one of the precarious wooden supports and clambered over the canvas. With nothing more than faith in the Almighty and the tensile strength of polyester, they've spray-painted a legend for the rest of their city to read in daylight: *MERCER RIP. CCS.*

I dig out the 35mm camera I stuffed into my denim jacket pocket earlier. Centring the graffiti, I marvel at the intensity of emotion that urged someone to dice with death for their artwork. I intend capturing the passions swirling around the stadium today and this madcap vandalism is the perfect opening salvo from the spool of 24. *1st click.*

Although it's a protest rally, the atmosphere feels like a cup tie. Fans stream towards the ground, brandishing green-white-green tricolours and saltires. Despite this scorching June afternoon, many are wearing the scarves they never for one moment thought they might be donning for the last time in 1990. An unruly bunch turn the corner into Easter Road in a straggling conga. *2ⁿᵈ click.*

*

Panning the crowds, I'm thinking of the highs and lows this club have taken their fans through. Zooming in on the tunnel I visualise the Famous Five appearing on match days. *3ʳᵈ click.* It's easy to imagine the roar sweeping around the terraces when Willie Ormond, Lawrie Reilly, Bobby Johnstone, Gordon Smith, and Eddie Turnbull emerged, the sunshine on Leith highlighting their Brylcreemed hair and the latter's forearm tattoo. A souvenir of Royal Naval Murmansk convoys.

That irony. A teenage Turnbull scanning the foreboding Arctic seas for periscopes. Becoming the first-ever British player to score in European competition when Hibs beat German champions, Rot-Weiss Essen in the 1955 European Cup, in a stadium rebuilt after being flattened by the RAF 10 years earlier.

This stadium has hosted many epic European encounters. A 3-2 defeat of Barcelona in the 1960-61 season, making an aggregate of 7-6. A 5-0 thumping of Napoli in 1967. After those highs, these past few weeks have represented the club's lowest ebb.

Picking out individual faces in the crowd, I take random shots. *4th click. 5th click.* I'll be on first name terms with many of them. Mates from Craiglockhart, scouts, Tynecastle, the punk scene, work, college. Neighbours from Shandon.

Now I'm tracking the Dunbar End, homing in on the different shirts. The red of Aberdeen and close by, what looks like an Arsenal shirt, red with white sleeves, except the North Londoners aren't sponsored by Forth Electrical Services. Stirling Albion. Behind, a knot of Hearts fans survey the segregation fences, getting used to cheers rather than abuse. *6th click.*

Segregation. Abuse. I'm reminded of one band practice, five years ago. We set up the amps and drum kit in Tom's flat in Leith Walk, by the Tommy Younger Bar (owned by the former goalie behind the Famous Five). Kenny shoved on the TV for the latest score of the European Cup final between Liverpool and Juventus. Riot police were clearing the Heysel Stadium terraces. Observing the confusing scenes from the commentary box, Jimmy Hill was suggesting National Service might solve England's perennial hooligan issues.

The camera zeroed in on fans wearing black and white. Amongst them, paramedics were working on someone's chest. A fan who'd saved up his wages and said goodbye to his family before travelling to Brussels from Turin to watch a football match. Now a stranger was fighting to bring him back to life.

I spot somebody wearing a faded Partick Thistle shirt, reminding me of Bradford City's claret and amber. *7th click.* Bradford, the Bantams, are my cousin Jimmy's second team.

Uncle Alex joined the Merchant Navy just before the war. Aged 15, he was so desperate to go to sea he threatened to run away from home if Grannie stood in his way. This situation prompted her to have a breakdown. She was hospitalised. (Although this was never discussed, she later confided in Anne she was bound in bandages due to her stress prompting extreme eczema – coupled with rapid weight loss she described herself 'resembling Gandhi.')

His ambition to sail the seven seas was the ultimate escape from Craigentinny, as far as possible from the factories and mills employing his father and neighbours. He would send exotic food parcels home, and at one point, during several days docked in Argentina, wrote to his mother enclosing a photograph of the stunning local girl he'd fallen for. A daughter of one of President Juan Perón's generals. After his Ben Line ship left Buenos Aires they lost touch.

By the 1960s he was ashore, married to an Edinburgh girl, rising through the ranks with Scottish Widows. He was promoted to a management post in Whitley Bay. His three sons, Jimmy, David and John became honorary Northumbrians. By the early 1970s, Jimmy and David were following Newcastle United across England, eager recruits of their feather-cutted, baggy trousered hooligan army.

When Uncle Alex was offered the position of Glasgow branch manager, the family uprooted back over the border, settling in Helensburgh. Even when involved in terracing skirmishes with a United scarf tied to one wrist, Jimmy always wore his ancestry like a badge of honour. In 1977 he swapped black and white for tartan, joining the thousands of Tartan Army foot soldiers swarming over Wembley and tearing down the goalposts after England 1 Scotland 2. A tiny chunk of that pitch was transplanted to my Auntie Marion's garden. The following year, Jimmy married a Yorkshire lass, Hilary, settling outside Bradford.

After flitting further south, one traumatic event was an occasion when Jimmy was interviewed by the police during the so-called Yorkshire Ripper case. This came in the wake of the notorious cassette sent to taunt the Assistant Chief Constable heading the manhunt, George Oldfield. Amongst the mountain of clues the West Yorkshire Police were grappling with, Jimmy ticked boxes. Working in a tool factory, he had ready access to hammers. His time in Whitley Bay had also given him a Geordie brogue. Alas, this was but one of so many dead ends during that investigation. The clue was in the title the press gave the recording's narrator, 'Wearside Jack.' The hoaxer had a Sunderland, not a Newcastle accent.

But the worst experience occurred five years ago. Bradford won promotion to the Second Division. Having secured the title the week before, there was a carnival atmosphere for their final game of the season, commencing with the presentation of the Third Division trophy. This being the club's first silverware since winning Division Three (North) over half a century before, the attendance of 11,000 was double the average. Jimmy was present with his brother-in-law.

During Third Division games, choosing a vantage point was never an issue. Jimmy, his in-laws, and their friends often sat in the main stand. This sun-baked afternoon they opted for the packed open terracing behind the goals. About a minute before half-time, fans were clambering over seating in the main stand. Jimmy's assumption was a brawl had broken out, either between the home crowd and visiting Lincoln City supporters, or Bantams fans amongst themselves. Then black smoke began belching from a portion of seating towards the rear, prompting a mass evacuation. Sixty seconds later, this had become an inferno.

Jimmy watched as hundreds decanted onto the pitch, younger fans waving their champions banners before the TV cameras while the stand was consumed by flames. This rickety Victorian structure, unaltered since its build in 1886, had been condemned that season. A combination of flammable bituminous roofing felt, wooden seating, and years of litter accumulation below the seats created a tinderbox. Council engineers had written to the club's owner warning of the risks; the stand was earmarked for demolition in the summer to make way for concrete seating and a steel roof.

During the conflagration, rather than scrambling over to the pitch, fans nearer the rear attempted to make their way back to the turnstiles. Impeded by tar-black smoke and a horrific rain of burning timbers and molten tarpaulin, they discovered these exits locked. Most of the 56 who died were recovered from these hellish dead-ends.

I recall the news footage. At one point the camera tracked an elderly man, his entire body wreathed in flames, walking away from the inferno, almost as if unaware of his predicament. He was pounced upon by a throng of spectators and police officers, smothered in jackets. A former mill worker, he later died of his injuries.

Bradford wasn't his side of the family's only narrow escape. Like Turnbull, Mum's eldest brother was at sea during the war, receiving the Atlantic and Burma Star medals. One time Uncle Alex was due to sail from Liverpool and set off on the first leg of a long journey by catching a train from Portobello Station. An air raid on Merseyside meant the tracks needed emergency repairs, delaying his arrival. By the time he made it to Liverpool Docks, his ship had departed. It was torpedoed in the Irish Sea.

A Heinkel's bomb aimer hitting a railway line after pressing a button from 20,000 feet in the night sky: surgical precision, or a fluke? Which part of Valley Parade to watch the championship celebrations from? After all the Liverpool ticket applications for last year's FA Cup semi-final, which turnstile number at Hillsborough?

Returning to this sun-bathed afternoon, Joe Baker is receiving a hero's adulation which he acknowledges by dropping to his knees to kiss the turf. I note how spritely he remains for the striker who scored 102 goals in 117 league games. *8ᵗʰ click.*

I sweep the east terracing. A silver-haired man who'll have been here for the glory days of three championships between 1948 and 1952 with Hugh Shaw at the helm. *9ᵗʰ click.* A lad in an Inspiral Carpets T-shirt, cartoon cows with spliffs above the legend 'cool as fuck.' 10th *click*. I track the kaleidoscope of colours in the Dunbar End. The royal blue of St Johnstone and a couple from Cowdenbeath. Morton and Hamilton Accies hoops. A trio wearing Queen's Park shirts. 11th *click*.

With the perspective of distance, I frame the shots to capture a bunch of local rivals together. Ayr United and Kilmarnock. Clyde and Clydebank. 12th *click*. Then an unimaginable sight in any other circumstance, two Celtic fans joking with their buddy in a Rangers shirt. 13th *click*. I'm reminded of shots I've seen of the Christmas Day Armistice in 1914, soldiers the same age as these guys, uniforms a patchwork of greys and khaki after they swapped hats or overcoats, beaming at the lens. Burying the hatchet. Hours from returning to their respective trenches to carry on the senseless slaughter.

There are Partick and Meadowbank Thistle fans, the amber combinations continuing beyond with Motherwell, Alloa Athletic, and Berwick Rangers. Clusters of Dundee United and Dundee devotees stand together. The participants receiving particular appreciation are the smattering of Hearts supporters who've broken ranks today.

Sometime later I snap Pat Stanton as his impassioned voice sounds across the PA. 14th *click*. The Proclaimers, sons of a Leith docker from the Henry Robb shipyards – another local institution swept away by market forces a few years ago – lead the crowd in 'You'll Never Walk Alone.' 15th *click*. Fans of every colour join in. Through my viewfinder I home in on faces, many invigorated by alcohol.

A TV crew are making their way along the terracing: an interviewer, a cameraman, and an accomplice wielding the boom microphone. After chatting with various individuals, they reach me. Shaking my hand, the interviewer tells me he's from STV. Footage from this event is going to be broadcast later, and he wants to ask questions, starting with why I'm here. Grateful at the opportunity to articulate my inner fervour, I take a breath.

Waving my hand towards the east terracing, I realise I'm clutching a full Red Stripe which slops overboard. I don't remember finishing the one crumpled by my Sambas. I explain.

Rangers fans would be the first to sign any petition if Celtic were facing extinction. His expression tells me he's sceptical about this. Based on a century of bitter rivalry, that statement does sound hollow. So I switch to regurgitating a quote from my mate Kenny, who'll be on the East terracing.

Sheffield United *need* Wednesday. West Ham *need* Millwall. Torino *need* Juventus. There's a difference between rivals who love to hate and bigots who just fucking hate. Torino. I ask him if he saw Joe Baker a minute ago? I conclude that clubs *need* rivals. Every Yin *needs* a Yang. Rivalries are the lifeblood of football.

He tells me that's enough for his film, and shakes my hand again, selecting his next target. Shrugging, I spark a fag, slug the warm lager. Was I making sense or confusing him with verbal diarrhoea? It's a question that seems to be cropping up with increasing regularity.

Yin and Yang. As if there's a zen-like quality to rivalries. Often nothing could be further from the truth. The most disturbing incidence of soccer violence I ever witnessed came after a league encounter at Parkhead in 1983, Davie Hay's managerial debut for the home side. Nobody was hurt. But as Alan and I made our way back to Queen Street station, red, white and blue-bedecked supporters started hurrying ahead, that adrenaline rush surging through the ranks the way it always does when something is kicking off. Fans were surrounding a car snared in the traffic jam. Punching its roof. Kicking the doors.

As we drew level I assumed it was full of Celtic supporters whose ill-advised shortcut had taken them into the path of the hordes streaming from the away end. But there were no colours evident. A moment after I clocked the alarmed expression of the female driver I noticed her clothing and the identical attire of her three passengers. They were nuns.

As well as the blows, salvos of spit were being aimed at the windows. Nothing like the way I'd witnessed the teenage sheep gobbing at punk bands taking the stage at Clouds. These were grown men, bellies swilling with beer, hacking up mouthfuls of vile sputum that was now clinging to the windscreen like the glop oozing from the creature's jaws in *Alien*. So much human venom had been coughed over the car, the terrified driver was forced to engage the wipers.

Some watched with revulsion, fathers stepping in front of their kids, shielding them from this, the far end of the wedge resulting from the club's historical 'traditions,' like spectators watching a Nuremberg book pyre with shame rather than exultation.

There were no physical injuries. But those Brides of Christ would now be bearing the mental scars of sectarianism. Adding to them, if they spent much time driving through Glasgow. I'm sure their cardinal Christian rule to forgive, non-existent amongst these 'Protestant' hate criminals, was tested. If I'd had a camera that day, I would have captured so many faces twisted by a nonsensical generation-spanning hatred not one of them could have explained, glaring into the steamed-up windows, their crass ignorance reflected.

Marx described religion as the opium of the people. Sectarianism, venal as heroin cut with rat poison, has been dividing and ruling the people for centuries.

52

Mass Hibsteria

The home crowd are pouring up towards London Road. *16ᵗʰ click.* My mishmash of colours provokes an occasional pantomime *hissssss* but mostly applause. Someone rushes over, seizes my hand. In his tearful eyes, I see passion. Community. Family ties. An entire subculture running parallel to yet divorced from machiavellian moneymaking schemes.

The Clan's shaded interior is a relief from the blazing sunshine, the nicotine-shrouded atmosphere rowdy. Roaring conversations. Hibs songs. Edging my way to the bar, I spy Kenny chatting to an older guy. Amidst the sea of football colours and 'Hands Off Hibs' T-shirts, conspicuous in a collar and tie. Grasping four Pils bottles, I make my way over. When I get closer I realise he's Ron Brown, Labour MP for Leith.

Kenny introduces us and we shake hands. By now I'm seeing everything through swimming vision. The skin around his face and neck seems disfigured. When Kenny adds the epithet *Red Ron*, Ron smiles, raising his glass in a mock toast.

That nickname is enough to dislodge tabloid stories from the back of my mind. I'm now drinking with someone the press label a firebrand, a loose cannon on his party's far-left, responsible for as many lurid headlines as quotes about his policies. He's one of the sharpest thorns in the side of the Thatcher administration, a presence in the Commons that The Speaker's eyes must drift towards with apprehension. A headache for his own party whips. You suspect he was the mouthy troublemaker at the back of his class in Ainslie Park, challenging his teacher's interpretation of Scotland's history. Forever framed in its British Imperial context.

I enquire about him being kicked out Parliament for throwing the Mace at someone. He snorts, sips his short. Explains how casting it onto the floor somehow caused over a grand's worth of damage. When Red Ron describes the red mist descending, his rising voice draws glances. I can see why Thatcher's front benches must bristle when he stands to speak. That combination of passion, eloquence and a working-class Scottish accent always arrests attention. Billy Connolly. Jimmy Reid. Red Ron. To my ears, it's poetic and beautiful.

At one point he heads off to the Gents. Weaving through the packed bodies, he looks so incongruous for someone taken to wielding the Mace in the Palace of Westminster. I'm reminded of that lone student on Tiananmen Square last year. Halting a tank column.

I mention how the Mace incident will make a brilliant piece for a concept album if we ever get round to any more recordings under the 'Leith Band Agnes' banner. An even bigger fan of The Fall than I am, Kenny once waxed lyrical about Mark E Smith writing the play 'Hey! Luciani,' about the mysterious death of John Paul the First. This ran for two weeks at the Riverside Studios in Hammersmith, and was described by Smith as a cross between Shakespeare and *The Prisoner*. Smith claimed he wrote the screenplay on beermats which he passed to the director in a shoebox.

Now I'm envisaging a script about the Mace, this implement being passed down the centuries like an Olympic baton. Defining Britain's often tenuous hold on democracy, commencing with Cromwell usurping the divine right of Kings only to turn Ireland into a bloodbath. All the way to Red Ron's stand against Thatcher. Against Mercer.

Kenny grins but can't disguise his caginess about this harebrained idea. Chinking his bottle against mine, he turns when a ponytailed lad wearing an Iggy Pop T-shirt accosts him, the Hibernian crest stamped on his forearm. His expression flares when he notices my scarf but warms when he clocks the 'Hands Off Hibs' stickers.

Gulping my Pils, I study the twin versions of that inked badge: the football, laurel leaves and crown I perfected from drawing them on school jotters. This recollection and the awareness of the blue, white and red material draped around my neck should've instilled a sense of regret. But alcohol and mania easily obliterate a conscience.

After Kenny breaks away from the conversation he asks about the flyers I mentioned. Delving into my jeans, I produce folded A4 sheets. Unfurling one, he grins at the incendiary content: *CCS. CSF. CSC. ASC. UTILITY. SECTION B. LOVE STREET DIVISION. SATURDAY SERVICE. ICF. CSS. You've united the factions you hate, Mercer. The crews and the fanzines. FUCK YOU.*

Kenny works at the Central Library. He tells me they get handed in copies of everything printed in Edinburgh, from flyers to LRT timetables to fanzines. My interest is sparked by the thought of a repository of punk zines. *Cripes. Cranked Up. Ripped and Torn.* He mentions a Hibs zine, *Mass Hibsteria*. One of his mates writes a lot of their stuff, a lad from Muirhouse called Irvine. His pieces are biting. And fucking hilarious. Kenny is forever telling Irvine he'll be a professional writer one day.

There's a dose of Meadowbank Thistle zines, for such a wee club. *Meadowbank Review. Cheers. The Thistle. AWOL.* John Peel's a huge fan and has even been to a few of their games. The Meadowbank fanzines are like a crossover with the punk zines. In-between printing merciless digs at their club's board, they write gig reviews and give away flexi singles.

I tell Kenny, on the way to The Clan I met a bloke who introduced himself as 'Square Goes' Christie, claiming to be the brother of the Meadowbank manager, Terry. He was carrying a massive holdall full of videos, hawking them at three for a tenner. I told him I was saving my beer vouchers.

Kenny explains everything handed into the library for classification gets its own catalogue number. If the worst comes to the worst, if there is ever a Hibs museum, my flyers would be added to the artefacts.

After joining us again, Ron shudders into his drink, murmuring how he wouldn't even want there to be a *Hearts* museum. The capital needs both clubs. *And* the old Ferranti Thistle.

Draining his glass, Ron hands it to me, asks me to pop it on the table. With an introspective smirk, he muses he doesn't want to end up in his wife May's bad books. *Again.* Winking, he shakes my hand. I notice scar tissue on his hands. He concludes by telling me it was a pleasure to meet someone wearing the Hillbilly Boy colours who was a Hibee at heart.

Kenny concurs with this sentiment, casting up a drunken party over in Tom's flat when I spent the entire evening draped in his Hibs scarf. Anyone else who sometimes travelled on the Union Jack bus touching green would've fucking melted. Like the Witch of the West of Scotland.

I tell them I'm a lone voice and if I ever go back on that bus the goading will be relentless. *Supporting the Leith Celtic must be down to your Royal Ed happy pills.*

Before Ron slips out, I request another portrait. Straightening his back, he raises his fist. I frame him, capturing flags in the background. Scottish saltire. Republic of Ireland tricolour. A maroon banner, context transforming its hated Heart of Midlothian logo into a potent symbol of Edinburgh working-class solidarity. *17ᵗʰ click.*

Wrapping an arm around Kenny, he assumes a more relaxed pose. I snap the pair, united by their love of Hibernian, their excessive grins belying the tension of the situation that has brought them here. *18ᵗʰ click.*

As he makes his way towards the door, I ask Kenny about Ron's scars. He explains Ron started off as a spark, like he did. He worked for Parsons Peebles but was in an accident. Took a hell of a belt. Needed extensive plastic surgery.

Moments after he's gone, a sonorous voice breaks into 'Sunshine on Leith,' title track of The Proclaimers second album and now Hibernian's unofficial anthem. Charged with emotion, its plaintive melodies surge like wildfire.

I spy a spare chair. Clambering onto it, Kenny keeps me balanced as I record the moment. *19ᵗʰ click. 20ᵗʰ click. 21ˢᵗ click.* Many of this impromptu choir are in floods of tears. As the chorus rings out, I'm 11 again. Oblivious to an unfathomable future, to the Sunday School picnic in two years time. Or incarceration in an intensive psychiatric care unit 13 years later. Giddy with anticipation. I've arrived at the uppermost steps on the main terracing for the first time. Dad's hand on my shoulder, butterflies swarming, I gawk into the arena, into the thousands upon thousands, the green and white scarf I've been wearing to school draped over my khaki-coloured parka. The atmosphere thick with unfamiliar nicotine. Mud on the tannoy. 'Tiger Feet.'

I accept I've no right to cling to these sentimental memories. Everyone else in my viewfinder would rather lose a limb than introduce the Govan bigots to their allegiances, with or without chemical imbalances. But at least I'm here.

I've never abandoned my childhood heroes and today's events have exposed the gulf between the team I loved as an innocent youngster, shy but full of beans as my Craiglockhart teacher Miss Mackenzie once wrote on a report card, and a Glasgow institution whose fans revel in their reviled status with battle chants like 'No One Likes Us, We Don't Care.'

Charlie and Craig Reid's lyrics might begin with a broken heart but they crescendo into a fierce expression of resilience and unabashed joy. Capturing these faces, I freeze these moments of unconditional love for club and community, finishing the remainder of the spool. *22nd click. 23rd click. 24th click.*

While the chief puts sunshine on Leith, how much longer will there be a stadium at Easter Road to be bathed in it? I feel my own tears.

53

35mm Dreams

There I am on STV, in my *deutsche* eagle zippy – as worn by many a Hoochie Coochie clubber (with *zero* far-right connotations) – and my scarf of many colours. Despite my rambled monologue to camera, I'm beaming with pride. Mum just frowns, notes I was captured smoking and said something that had to be bleeped. Crestfallen, I retreat to my room. But nothing can dampen my emotions. Today's events seemed like an extrapolation of Ron's multifaceted human rights struggles.

I rummage around bottom drawers and the detritus cluttering wardrobes, digging out creased Hibs programs that cost 5p, unfurling the *Evening News* souvenir poster of the 1972 League Cup win. The sight of that yellowing, creased poster makes me maudlin. But I'm also inspired. Sitting in front of my typewriter, I compose an intro to my photography book.

FOOTBALL SEGREGATES PEOPLE BUT ITS GREATEST PROP-
ERTY IS ITS CAPACITY TO UNITE. CAN YOU IMAGINE THE
CHRISTMAS TRUCE IN 1914 WITH THE TOMMIES TRUDGING
OVER NO MAN'S LAND WITH BADMINTON RACKETS?

MY OWN RELATIONSHIP WITH THE BEAUTIFUL GAME HAS
BEEN HOT AND COLD. CONTRADICTORY. AMBIVALENT. MIXED
UP. BUT WHAT IS CAST IRON IS MY EMPATHY WITH THE
SENSE OF OUTRAGE AT WHAT IS HAPPENING TO HIBS, A CLUB
EMBEDDED IN THE LEITH AND EDINBURGH COMMUNITIES FOR
115 YEARS.

MERCER'S BID TO EXPLOIT HIBERNIAN AS A MEANS TO
IMPROVE HIS SHARE PORTFOLIO IS A MICROCOSM OF THE
WAY THATCHERISM HAS ORDERED HUGE SWATHES OF SCOT-
LAND'S INDUSTRIAL HEARTLAND, THE HOI POLLOI SHE AND
HER LACKEYS ARE SO SCORNFUL OF, TO BE SWEPT ASIDE
WHENEVER THEY ARE NO LONGER DEEMED PROFITABLE.

Dad pokes his head around the door and suggests any overtime I'll be earning this month will already have been blown in
the pub. Shaking my head at this, I go into a rant about how
inspiring the rally was, and meeting Ron Brown MP. How I've
preserved the fantastic occasion for posterity. The poignancy
of rivals uniting. How my photos will be worth their weight in
gold and I'm *seriously* going to get into photography. Escape
from the Scottish Office. How I'm going to publish a book
about it all. *Hands Off Hibs*. Portrait of a club's fight for
survival. Portrait of a club's last stand?'

He listens with scepticism. But he was an enthusiastic amateur photographer at my age. He asks where the camera is: it was his trusty Kodak 35mm camera I borrowed. Over the decades he created hundreds of precious memories with it, even setting up a darkroom to develop his negatives and create enlargements in the old coal cellar beneath the stairs. Anne and I were too young to appreciate the gravity of the 'Do Not Disturb' sign affixed to the door, would barge inside and ruin the occasional spool. He tells me he'll unwind the film since this can be tricky. Then I can take the cartridge in to get developed next week.

After he exits, I shove my headphones on and flip the Stereo MCs onto the turntable. *33-45-78*. I caught them at Calton Studios last October, supporting A Certain Ratio. They came close, but not quite, to blowing Manchester's finest funkateers off the stage. I was so inspired I bought this album from the merch stall. Cranking up the volume I nod in time to the furious rhythm. I sing along. *We ain't hooligans on a football pitch.* I pounce on the typewriter keys again.

HIBERNIAN MAY HAVE BEEN BORN IN THE COWGATE BUT THEY HAVE BEEN PART OF THE FABRIC OF LEITH SINCE THE 1890S; THE SAME LEITH THAT VOTED FIVE TO ONE AGAINST MERGING WITH EDINBURGH IN 1920, A MERGER THAT WENT AHEAD WITH A CAVALIER DISREGARD FOR DEMOCRACY. MERCER, LIKE THATCHER, MIGHT BE A CHAMPION OF THE FREE MARKET BUT JUST AS THATCHER DECLARED THERE WAS NO SUCH THING AS SOCIETY, MERCER'S FAILURE TO RECOGNISE

THE PASSION OF HIBERNIAN'S FANBASE, EXEMPLIFIED BY THE TENS OF THOUSANDS WHO ATTENDED TODAY'S RALLY, REVEALS A SIMILAR DETACHMENT. MERCER ASSUMED HIS HOSTILE TAKE-OVER WAS ALL ABOUT ATTAINING THE MAGICAL FIGURE OF 76% OF THE CLUB'S SHARES, NOTHING MORE THAN THAT. HIS SPREADSHEETS AND FINANCIAL PROJECTIONS NEVER AC-COUNTED FOR THE FERVOUR OF AN ENTIRE COMMUNITY, GALVA-NISED BY THE HANDS OFF HIBS CAMPAIGN. THE FACT THE MOVEMENT'S FIRST DONATION WAS A GENEROUS CHEQUE FROM AN ANONYMOUS HEARTS FAN SPEAKS VOLUMES ABOUT THE GULF BETWEEN THE TERRACES AND BOARDROOMS.

TODAY HAS PROVED TO SCOTLAND AND THE WORLD THAT FOOTBALL HAS A MEANING FAR BEYOND THE LOWLY STATUS IT IS HELD IN BY STRANDS OF SOCIETY WHO LOOK DOWN ON ANY-THING THAT ISN'T TO DO WITH THEIR ENTITLEMENT. FOOTBALL HAS BEEN ENTHRALLING EVERYDAY PEOPLE FOR GENERATIONS, PEOPLE FOR WHOM AIRS AND GRACES ARE AS ALIEN AS GOOSE-STEPPING.

AND THERE HAS NEVER BEEN OR EVER WILL BE ANYTHING LIKE HILLSBOROUGH, VALLEY PARADE OR IBROX AT WIMBLEDON, THE OVAL OR TWICKENHAM.

A sub-text. When they're developed, I'll check my photos for any Liverpool shirts. Liverpool. Bradford City. Rangers. 96. 56. 66. There was also Bolton v Stoke in 1946. 33. Scotland v England at Ibrox in 1902. 25.

I'm thinking of the sea of green and white on three sides of the stadium, the multicoloured fourth. Should I match the

Dunbar End portraits according to palette? Aberdeen with Stirling Albion. Partick Thistle, Albion Rovers, and Meadowbank Thistle? Or geographically? Hibs to Meadowbank to Hearts, ever westwards, through Motherwell and Airdrie, onto Glasgow and Ayrshire, up to Greenock Morton, Dumbarton.

When my book is published to massive acclaim, I'll donate a percentage to the *Hands Off Hibs* campaign. But what percentage? Depends if it becomes a bestseller. Of course it will be.

Recalling my chat with Red Ron, I dig into the rear pockets of my 501s, tug out notes I scrawled onto a beermat, together with the biro Ron gave me. When I asked if he had a pen I could borrow, he gave me this souvenir, complete with the House of Commons portcullis crest. Although he added he preferred answering correspondence from constituents on headed paper. Not beermats.

I hold the torn cardboard up to the light. My transcription of his spiel is so frayed I might as well be an archaeologist with the first Sanskrit tablet unearthed by Indian villagers. But I can decipher snippets. Enough to seed my fertile mind. I start transcribing.

BROWN DESCRIBED THE POLL TAX AS A CLASS TAX. THATCHER WAS USING SCOTLAND AS ITS TESTING GROUND. WHEN THE POLL TAX IS ROLLED OUT TO THE REST OF THE UK, HER ROYAL HIGHNESS WILL PAY THE SAME TAX AS HER CLEANERS.

THATCHER ALSO SAID THE PROBLEM WITH SOCIALISM WAS RUNNING OUT OF OTHER PEOPLE'S MONEY. BROWN'S RIPOSTE

TO THAT WAS THAT THIS SO-CALLED OTHER PEOPLE'S MONEY
HAD TO COME FROM SOMEWHERE IN THE FIRST PLACE. AND
WHERE IT CAME FROM WAS OTHER PEOPLE'S TOIL AND SWEAT.
FOR CENTURIES. WHO BECAME RICH FROM EXPLOITING THE
WORKFORCE IN THE FACTORIES, THE MINES, THE SHIPYARDS
THAT FUELLED THE INDUSTRIAL REVOLUTION? AND WHO DIED IN
APPALLING CONDITIONS LONG BEFORE THE DAYS OF TRADE
UNIONS, WHEN INDUSTRIAL INJURIES WOULD LEAVE FAMILIES
DESTITUTE, CONSIGNING WOMEN AND CHILDREN TO WORK-
HOUSES?

AFTER SWEARING AN OATH TO SOME MONARCH FROM A
GERMAN ROYAL LINE, WHO DIED ON FOREIGN BATTLEFIELDS,
DISPROPORTIONATELY SCOTTISH AND IRISH? WHO COMPRISED
THE EMPIRE'S CANNON FODDER? NOT THE UPPER CLASSES, THE
LANDED GENTRY OR THE INDUSTRIAL BARONS.

AND WHAT ABOUT THE EMPIRE? BUILT ON SLAVERY, FAMINE
IN INDIA AND IRELAND, GENOCIDE IN AUSTRALIA. OTHER
PEOPLE'S MONEY? WHAT ABOUT OTHER PEOPLE'S BLOOD?

The next beermat is to do with Ron's Afghanistan trip but this
is lager-stained.

BROWN MET PRESIDENT KARMAL IN 1981, WHILE CARTER
WAS ORDERING THE CIA TO HAND BILLIONS TO JIHADISTS TO
FIGHT THE SOVIETS. THE JIHADISTS OPPOSED WOMEN'S RIGHT
TO EDUCATION. US STINGER MISSILES TARGETED SCHOOLS. MI6
ORGANISED COVERT OPS WITH THE MUJAHIDEEN.

THE CIA SIPHONED BILLIONS TO SADDAM DURING THE IRAQ
IRAN WAR. CHEMICAL WEAPONS WERE USED AGAINST IRANIANS
AFTER US SATELLITE FOOTAGE PINPOINTED AN ATTACK ACROSS
THE MESOPOTAMIAN MARSHES.
   SHIAS IN IRAN. AFGHAN SUNNIS. IRAQI SHIA AND SUNNI?
PICKING SIDES IS MADNESS. BIGGER PROBLEMS ONE DAY.

And as far as *The Sun* is concerned, Ron's main contribution to political history has been vandalising an ornament.

I start when the volume is killed. Dad is hovering over the record player. *There was no film in the fecking camera.* When the door closes I wrench the sheet from the typewriter, crumple it into the bin. It could've been worse. I could've assumed there were 36 in the spool.

My mind drifts to all the faces who gazed into the lens, assuming their stand this afternoon was being captured for posterity. Immortalised. So many colours, each representing respective stories. Promotion. Relegation. Names inscribed in silverware. Or destined never to be carved into any major trophy, a fact that diminished the intensity of that passion not one iota.

My eyes are teary again. I think of history's most poignant football match, between khaki and grey-clad opponents during the Christmas truce on the Western Front. Many of the participants gained immortality four years later, their names carved in stone, joining millions of similar inscriptions in Britain, France, Germany, Russia, America, Italy, the Balkans. Each one a son, father, husband, brother, cousin, uncle.

I tear up the beermats. Toss the shards into the air. They drift over the floor like the white feathers mailed by citizens from the comfort of their homes to neighbours to shame them into signing up for the King's Shilling. Dwelling on war, I'm reminded of something Mum and Dad once bemoaned.

Dad's first Hogmanay in his adopted home. Compared to recent experiences in Ireland, where the stroke of midnight prompted a perfunctory toast during a card game, the drinking and dancing that lasted through the night in Craigentinny was a joyous eye-opener.

Less welcome was being roused the following day to throw his dishevelled suit back on and clamber aboard a Gorgie-bound tram for the impending Ne'er Day Derby. Mum was also press-ganged by her older brother, Alex, home on leave.

Never interested in football, despite four of Hibernian's Famous Five performing at the peak of their abilities on the sleet-lashed pitch (and Hibs chasing their second league title in three years), my parents huddled on the packed terracing, seeking solace in Dad's hip flask. Neither remembered the result (2-1 to Hearts, Gordon Smith scoring a consolation goal four minutes from time). What most stuck in Mum's mind were instances when the St John's Ambulancemen were summoned to help fans who had collapsed with drink and injured themselves. Their mates would wave a white handkerchief.

This was 1951, only six years after the end of the war, so the universal signal of surrender would still be prominent in popular culture. Dad joked about spending most of the interminable 90 minutes on the verge of brandishing a hankie himself.

Another memory. At Napier College, our history professor, Ian Wood gave one lecture about sectarianism in Scottish football, focusing on the Old Firm, then discussing the Ibrox disasters of 1961 and 1971. His affable tones belied a narrative that chilled me to the bone.

He described fans decanting from Glasgow's vast Victorian-built bowls, Hampden, Ibrox, and Parkhead on matchdays, upwards of 80,000 spectators filtering down narrow, crumbling stairwells towards the few exits. At Ibrox, these stairways were precarious, their dirt steps trodden over by millions over the decades, the wooden rims exposed in many places to become booby traps. On one of these, stairway 13, a mass crush resulted after Jim Baxter scored a last-gasp equaliser during an Old Firm encounter in September 1961, prompting jubilant fans to collide on the dilapidated stairs. Two died. George Nelson and Thomas Thomson. But those events were eclipsed on Saturday, January 2nd 1971.

After a mediocre contest, most fans were anticipating returning to families or the pub, many already streaming towards the exits to avoid the customary overcrowding. But a roar erupted from the away end when Jimmy Johnstone found the net in the 89th minute. The green and white hordes were still cheering when Rangers were awarded a free kick. With the last kick of the game, Colin Stein equalised.

The home fans erupted, leaping from the ground, tossing scarves in the air. As those facing the other way turned, joining in the delirious celebrations, shockwaves surged through bodies already funnelling down stairway 13. A terrible momentum flowed through this seething tide of humanity, many unable to touch the steps with their feet. Thousands pressed on in a tsunami of red, white and blue, their weight buckling the metal handrails running down the centre of the stairwell. The triumphal chants swirling from the terraces drowning the increasing cries of anguish, the first of a flurry of white hankies were raised above the panic-stricken crowds. Sixty-six people died of suffocation, including five schoolmates from Markinch in Fife.

An accident waiting to happen, was how Ian summarised that afternoon's harrowing events. In what other walk of life other than football would a potential horror hanging over tens of thousands, week-in, week-out, have prompted such a *laissez-faire* attitude from the government and sports authorities?

The youngest victim, Nigel Pickup, was only in Scotland for the New Year and had been taken to his first and last match by a family friend. Aged eight, he was from Prescot outside Liverpool, another city forever associated with the needless, preventable deaths of fans who'd gone to watch a game of football and never come home.

Clawing the paper fragments I crumple them into the bucket. The thought of taking my lighter to it all flits through my mind. Instead, I lie down, facing the ground like Joe Baker did while the sun shone on Leith, before twisting around, gazing into the ceiling tiles. Losing myself in the music's relentless beat.

54

Commandos And
Playwrights

Arms folded, I scowl out the windscreen. Two and a half years have passed since the acute breakdown that led to me being sectioned. I hoped that would be a once-in-a-lifetime experience of a psychiatric unit. Now, on a cracking summer's afternoon, youngsters heading towards the Meadows with footballs to emulate Andy Roxburgh's *Italia 90* squad, I'm being driven to the Royal Edinburgh Hospital again. Anne in the back seat for moral support.

Making another plea, I insist there's nothing wrong with me. If I seem excitable it's because I *am* excited. If I appear to be high it's because I'm high on life. Everything's happening at once. It's an *exciting time* for me just now. I blurt out the shortlist of these exciting things, again, although the list is anything but short.

There's the new job. A *permanent* job, albeit with the conditional proviso. The probational clause based on my underlying health condition. But that's just so much Scottish Office red tape. My manic condition is ancient history. There's the new flat. There's the Madchester music scene, a glorious collision of rock and house: The Stone Roses spattered in paint in posters on my bedroom wall, The Inspiral Carpets 'This is How it Feels' taped from *Top of the Pops* last week, *The Stone Roses* album, Happy Mondays 'Wrote For Luck' and 'Step On,' and The Charlatans new single, 'The Only One I Know,' all on constant rotation on my turntable. There's Scotland in the World Cup for the fifth time on the bounce.

When I went to college after almost four years in the Widows, I never moved into digs. Napier was close enough to go home for lunch. Now I'm making up for lost time.

Freedom, I reiterate. You were young once, Dad.

Anne sniggers but I'm getting this vibe from him. Part irritation. Mostly concern. He says when he overhears me on the phone these days, my constant chatter reminds him of Robin Williams in *Good Morning, Vietnam*. Nothing wrong with being verbose. But there *is* when it's so opposite to my normal personality.

I counter this by demanding he define *normal*. So he goes on about how it's *abnormal* to have started accosting neighbours. *And* strangers. *Assailing* them with my monologues. What was I even saying to Mr Brown at number 7 the other day?

I explain about Mr Brown. During the war, he was a commando. I was telling him I could ghostwrite his life story. He'll have *spellbinding* memories. Most people's impression of war comes from cinema. TV. *Dad's Army* is never off the box. A world where the Nazis were an all-pervasive threat that finally materialised when a captured U-Boat captain took names for the firing squads. The guy that played Godfrey, Arnold Ridley, that sweet old gentleman who was either enthusing about his sisters Sissy and Dolly's fairy cakes or asking to be excused. He experienced hand-to-hand fighting at the Somme. I read about him in a book about the making of *Dad's Army*. Ridley went over the top with the Somerset Light Infantry. Twice. The second time he discovered an enemy trench unmarked on the reconnaissance map. With many of his comrades scythed by surprise machine gun fire, he worked his way along this trench, lobbing grenades. Got whacked over the head by a German's rifle butt. Deflected a bayonet lunge away from his stomach, but into his groin. His left wrist was also lacerated by a bayonet strike. After the war, he underwent 15 operations to try and save his hand. Three fingers remained numb. Numb, like a spot on my right knee struck by a log at a scout camp in Bonaly.

Poised to go off on that tangent, I rein myself in. The other day Anne bemoaned my erratic chatter. After enquiring about eligible single girls from her office, I somehow ended up explaining I was going to paint the album cover of *The Dark Side of The Moon* over the tent a guy at work, Chris was taking to Glastonbury. He said last year there were unofficial sound systems all over the site, churning out acid house 24/7. Chris, a prog fan, is also into techno. He gave me a cassette of The Orb on John Peel last December. They're dancey. But trippy. They did one 20-minute track for the whole session like Wire did back in 1979. 'Crazy about Love.' Broadcast the Tuesday after the September weekend. The day I started working full-time.

But I try sticking to my current theme. If you look close enough you can spot Ridley's awkward left-hand movements. He also experienced regular blackouts as a result of his cracked skull. Lived in fear of collapsing on stage. War has always been sanitised. Only combatants have the remotest idea of what it's like. The biggest trauma I've faced lately was nicking my finger when I was slicing cheese with a bread knife. Imagine witnessing your best mates' guts splattered over a muddy field after some general added an arrow to Somerset Light Infantry on a map? A dodgy map. I get the poppies. Why it's so important to remember the people behind the millions of names carved into white crosses. But beyond all those names and serial numbers of lads, like Mum's grandad, who died for King and Country? Someone's loved one being murdered in ways *nobody* can imagine. Obliterated by industrially-produced shells. Asphyxiated by chlorine gas. Gored by bayonets. Drowned in oceans of mud.

Something else I read. The majority of deaths weren't even during battle. They were through influenza. Pneumonia. Trench fever. Soldiers lived among rotting corpses of men and horses. Each man's death would be the starting pistol for a feeding frenzy. Rats. Worms. Microbes. I'm reminded of 'Reuters,' the opening track on Wire's brilliant *Pink Flag* debut.

Casualties increasing... enemy shellfire... Flies and rats thriving... Without the lifetime shield of immune systems, bacteria would run riot. By the trillions. Another book I'm reading...

Which one, interrupts Dad. Reminds me I leave opened books all over the place these days. He found one under the settee about the Swinging Sixties.

That. I ask if either of them has heard of Stuart Sutcliffe? Blank expressions. I explain he was The Beatles' first bassist, co-inventing their name with John Lennon. He left them to focus on his art before they became famous. Although he was a quiet lad, his paintings were intense. Dark. He was from Edinburgh. I've only heard of him cause Adam Ant namechecks him in his song, Friends.

Anne asks if *he* ever became famous, through his art? Alas, no. He *was* talented. But he received a head injury when he was attacked outside a club in Liverpool after one of their early gigs, in 1961. *His* skull was cracked, just like Arnold. Lennon broke a finger in the fracas. After that, Stuart was plagued by headaches. Died of an aneurysm the following April, aged 21. Lennon would still refer to him as his alter-ego. His spirit guide. Displayed some of his paintings. He's also immortalised on the cover of Sergeant Pepper. A quiet lad from Edinburgh, with hidden depths?

Before either can respond, I go back to the book I wanted to discuss. About the origins of the Great War. The war to end all wars. All those Germans dying for the Kaiser? And the British and Commonwealth troops dying for the King? The Kaiser's mother was Vicky, Victoria's eldest daughter. Kaiser Wilhelm

II, King George V, and Tsar Nicholas II were cousins, all three direct descendants of King George II, from Hanover. George and Tsar Nicholas's mothers were sisters from the Danish royal family. Didn't prevent George from refusing him exile, then shifting the blame for his decision onto Lloyd George when the Tsar, Tsarina, and their five children were slaughtered. Queen Victoria meddled in the love lives of her 42 grandchildren. Arranging matches. Ensuring her bloodline bound Europe's monarchies. Instead, Europe, with its inbred ruling classes, was consumed by a bloodbath that decimated each country's lower classes. *That's* mental.

Dad's lips are pursed while a driver takes an age reversing the 4x4 from his driveway.

Backtracking to John Brown's biopic I mention *bestseller* in this context but regret it. That's what I've been stating about several book ideas. I retrieve the upper hand by mentioning May Annandale. Teenagers passing the woman from number 1 Briarbank Terrace at the Shandon shops only see a white-haired old lady. Without kids of her own, she would spoil Anne and me, baking birthday cakes and Easter cakes decorated with tiny chocolate eggs and ornamental chicks. She knitted me a green and white bobble hat. But when May was younger than I am now, she was in the Royal Army Nursing Corps. One of the first nurses who entered Bergen-Belsen concentration camp following liberation in April 1945. I emphasise the poignancy of this by revealing something I read the other day. Some survey of attitudes of under-25s. Half the respondents didn't know who died in the Holocaust.

Anne asks if Mr Brown is going to take me up on my offer? I tell her, *maybe*.

Probably not, Dad observes. Some people deal with the horrors they've seen by *burying* the memories. That's how they cope. He concludes I've probably unnerved the poor guy.

Unnerved. I scoff at that. Someone who was parachuted behind German lines when he was a teenager?

Dad asks me to put myself in Mr Brown's shoes. All his life he's known a shy boy, maybe with some outlandish teenage fashions. All of a sudden this lad's accosting him on his doorstep.

Would he rather I behaved like a Stepford Wife? Or at least, one of their sons? Son of a Stepford Wife? Stepford Wife and Son. Here I emphasise the pun I'm grasping for by whistling the *Steptoe and Son* theme, tapping the dashboard.

Now he reiterates how manic I seem. He's been reading up about it. My mental condition has regressed beyond hypomania, a daily lapse, to mania, more drawn-out behaviour. He says this is just as scary to everyone in the family as when I was ill three years ago when I *wouldn't* talk. It's as if I'm high all the time. *Am I high* a lot of the time?

Not *all* the time. But I regret being so flippant. Alluding to recreational drugs will harm my defence. I add a flourishing key change to my shrill refrain, remembering the door-to-door insurance man back in the 1960s. He would whistle his way up and down the stairs like a skylark. Winking when he caught sight of me or my sister.

Concluding the troubling exchange, Dad says this interview is just a precaution. I clam again, not wanting to appear *manic*.

We're turning into the car park. I feel so distant from the person who was locked up in the Intensive Psychiatric Care Unit. Those memories almost seems implanted, a common enough science fiction trope. *Total Recall*. But the setting is so recognisable.

55

Touching 10

When Dr Grant strolls into the waiting area, I spring from the seat I've been slouched in. Demand to be seen on my own. The psychiatrist peers at Dad. They exchange conspiratorial nods. Following the doctor into his office, I drag the chair opposite his desk into place, then slump, arms across my chest. Dr Grant informs me Dad explained what's been going on in a somewhat distressed phone call earlier.

He *grassed* on me? I'm indignant. Dr Grant remains professional. He stresses the root of my parents' concerns is their worry I'm approaching another breakdown. Whether bipolar cycles soar or crash, the outcome is unhealthy. He asks me to describe how I've been feeling.

Relieved about this opportunity to explain everything to someone who'll understand, I launch into a spiel. The new job. The music. The football. Moving away from home into a flat in Dalry to become my wee sister's lodger.

I try lightening the mood by announcing I'm now free to invite girls back for a *coffee*. Adding air quotes. I know there's so much more I want to fill him in on. Stuff that will illustrate why this is all about excitement. A *lust for life*. Maybe not allude to Iggy Pop. Barechested Godfather of punk and the world's first stage diver. Mania as rock 'n' roll performance.

I'll try applying a filter. If I become too talkative he'll collude with that farcical *manic* hypothesis. A good mood. Feeling positive. Not the same as *manic*. No way.

So what if I'm chattier than everyone who knows me are all used to? *Fuck them all*. I *think* that. Prevent myself from blurting it out. Although I notice that despite my constraint, his biro is *flowing* across the lines of his notepad. Is he scrutinising my body language? He'll know more than most how 90% of all communication is nonverbal. I stop fidgeting.

Force myself to sit still. Cross my legs. I was chewing my gum like a football manager, so I clam my jaws. Lucidity is the way to go. If I can demonstrate I'm in full control of my glowing emotions, no one can use those snide two syllables. *Manic*. My arse. I've discovered I *like* chatting, Dr Grant. This time I'm thinking this *and* telling him. I ponder expanding on this with examples. Explaining about meeting a new mate in the pub. I'll remain calm as I describe this. *Lucid*.

Martin's from Londonderry. Or Derry. Depending. The city's electoral boundaries are the dictionary definition of *gerrymandering*. Split into one large Catholic district, the South Ward, where nationalist voters outweigh unionists by ten thousand to one thousand, and two smaller areas, North and Waterside Wards, where unionists outvote nationalists by a couple of thousand. The result: unionist-controlled city councils. Although these notions are whizzing through my mind, I keep them in check.

Whighams Wine Bar after the football. I overheard Martin's accent. I butted in. Told him my old man was from Monaghan. He frowned. But moved to Fermanagh. That hop over the border was enough to restore his smile.

Edinburgh Uni student. We ended up chatting for ages. About the Troubles. About Northern Ireland being defined by them although there are more murders per annum in Strathclyde. About the Federation of Conservative Students. Martin's an FCS organizer. Edinburgh branch. Opposing the National Union of Students. Unlikely as it might have been for someone known as diffident his whole life, with a father who has always favoured Irish unity and a lifelong socialist mother, we clicked. Became buddies. Socialising. He introduced me to bars where the FCS hung out. Glaring at the Tory Wets in their floppy *Brideshead Revisited* fringes, Pringle sweaters around their shoulders.

Not a mate as in Grum or Alex, longstanding friendships cultivated through a shared love of punk and countless lost weekends of drunken adventures. Martin mistook my manic side... *excitement*... as an indication of an affable extrovert who seemed genuine in engaging with his unionist politics. But I was just as enthusiastic after meeting two Mormons earlier in the summer. They showed up at Mum and Dad's. I asked them in for coffee. *No*, they didn't drink coffee. *Off-limits* according to their teachings. But they accepted water.

So I brought these two besuited men, around my age, speaking in US Midwestern drawls, glasses of water. Accepted a videotape from them which the three of us became engrossed in until Dad crashed into the room, stabbed the eject switch, demanded they legged it. Like Jesus ejecting the moneylenders. I was both mortified and relieved to see the back of them and their weird propaganda.

Lucidity? I could give Dr Grant my objective appraisal of Martin's oddness after I invited him round to Anne's flat to chill out. He *did* accept a coffee. Every Christian sect has a different interpretation of the rules in their ancient book.

Anne was also entertaining her pal, Laura. Martin's first whispered question to me about Laura? Not the obvious one, *is she single?* It was *is she a fenian?* He said it just like that. So matter of fact. As if it's what constitutes an icebreaker where he's from. Course it is. That's how they decide which football team to support. How elections are rigged. *Is she a fenian?* That F-word. Ulster's answer to the N-word in Mississippi.

His cherrypicking of his homeland's history was as unrefined as Derry's biased suffrage. To him, William of Orange was the folk hero on the gable ends. Forever crossing the River Boyne on his resplendent white charger. Redacted from Martin's narrative was the fact King Billy was supported by Pope Innocent XI because that 1690 battle was one encounter during a wider European conflict, the Nine Years War, or War of the Grand Alliance. The Grand Alliance being England, Holland, Spain, Portugal *and* the Holy Roman Empire, versus France.

Also absent from his dogmatic mindset would be the Irish Famine of 1740. The Great Hunger of 1845. The 1798 rebellion that allied Protestants and Catholics as United Irishmen against the Anglican establishment, an uprising characterised by wholescale massacres of civilians, of whom the Ulster Presbyterians suffered the greatest repression at the hands of redcoats.

I'll maybe tell Dr Grant how Martin thought I was so lucid I'd make an excellent spokesman for the FCS. The FCS model themselves on soccer boys. Call themselves *Maggie's Millwall.* Instead of impassioned debates with Labour students, they just steam into their meetings. Like politics in 1930s Germany. The FCS have their own newspaper. *Capitalist Worker.* Martin said they sell it wherever they see someone standing on a corner selling *Socialist Worker.* They stand in front of them. Noising them up. If the red says anything he gets a fat lip.

I was supposed to have a meeting with Martin and some of his colleagues. But I forgot which pub. I think I got the time wrong, too. Just as well. Cause they sounded like a bunch of middle-class bullies. The whole bluenose thing might've been a weird front for me, ill-fitting with my genuine allegiances. But nowhere near as incongruous as championing Far-Right students. But. Martin is affable. Easy to chat to. We're both into The Charlatans.

A couple of weeks ago, I popped up to his flat for a coffee and catch up. He stuck 'The Only One I Know' onto his record player. Started freaking out, swinging his arms. Though I was sober as a judge, I joined in. Music can do that. Kill inhibitions. Shame it couldn't do the same to his politics.

I find it so easy to make new mates these days. But I can also recognise Martin's mindset is the result of centuries of political volatility. Of history distorted and spun. In no other corner of Britain are young minds so ripe for polarisation. While I'm pondering whether to articulate my whirring thoughts, Dr Grant's pen has continued its remorseless flow. He flips over a page.

Something Dad once told me. His father, for all his unionism and a job as a caretaker at a Masonic Hall in Enniskillen, was once held at gunpoint by Black and Tans. Churchill's thugs, terrorising everyone they saw as *micks*. The Tans were recruited from unemployed Great War veterans at the same time Hitler was mobilising his Brownshirts. Irish independence's greatest recruiting sergeants.

Dad's view of Irishness is always romantic rather than political, other than the biggest political viewpoint of all: that Ireland should never have been carved up by the British Empire, its artificial border based on nothing more than a sectarian headcount. Dad's Ireland isn't 17th-century battles or drums. It's Oscar Wilde. W.B. Yeats' poetry. But not his Blueshirt sympathies. The Irishmen who fought for Franco. As bad as Irishmen fighting Irishmen for England.

Most of all, the songs he loves singing when he's drinking Carlsberg Special. The mountains of Mourne sweeping down to the sea... The sun going down on Galway Bay... Never, *ever* about being up to his knees in fenian blood.

Unlike the cretins who dip into sectarianism's malevolence, whether from a football terrace or to exclude candidates from job vacancies, Dad experienced its reality.

I once came across a yellowing certificate. His Orange Lodge membership. When I asked about this, he admitted this memento was a keepsake from his youth. Nothing more. He abandoned the ridiculous Ulster/Ireland schism decades ago when his little brother, Jim fell in love with a Catholic. Their father asked Dad to implore Jim to finish this relationship. Dad, ever the hopeless romantic, respected the course of true love more than hate. My paternal grandfather's blinkered religious intolerance was exposed in stark relief. Dad refused any *intervention*. Uncle Jim joined the Post Office on the mainland, as Dad had done. Settled in Swindon with the girl who became my Auntie Sheila. They brought up their two daughters, Caroline and Sue, my English cousins, free of his homeland's insane enmity. Dad went even further, claiming the source of all Ireland's problems could be summarised in one word. England.

Mentioning Martin in the context of positivity and excitement and *lucidity* could be misconstrued as manic. So I consign the thought to the back burner. Ireland. Religion. *Off-limits* when you're pleading innocence of manic outbursts to a psychiatrist.

I want to let the doctor see I can place my illness in perspective. Anyone's life can alter in the most transient of moments. For me, it hinged on one phone call. Inviting me to a Sunday School picnic. I could've just ignored that bleating, *bleating*, bleating sound eating into my eardrums. Had I done so, I might not be here today.

When I think of this irony of alternative scenarios, my fertile imagination pictures the Serb activist who assassinated an Austro-Hungarian Archduke. Only because Franz Ferdinand's chauffeur took a wrong turning and halted outside the café where his killer happened to be sitting. Within four years, 40 million people had died. How many millions upon millions of fatherless British, German, French, Russian, Austrian, Serbian, Italian children? Down to happenstance.

My eyes are drawn to a swallow fluttering around the eaves outside. But I won't get distracted. When my train of thought is hurtling like this, it gets derailed. I try articulating my Sarajevo moment happened in the summer of 1976. Except I'm astute enough to filter out 'Sarajevo.' My moment, when the seeds were sown that would unspool in 1987, was the day I was abused, an event I blame for leaving such an indelible stain on my psyche.

Dr Grant nods at this and scribbles something else down. He concurs environmental factors can be a potent trigger for bipolar disorder. Stress. Bereavement. *Abuse*. In this context, mental *injury* rather than illness would the more appropriate description.

I consider steering away from the conjecture of what might have contributed to my mental instability. I must remain *lucid*. Maybe talk about music again. I've *always* loved music, from hearing The Beatles on the radio as a kid to my own band being played on Radio 1. Music led me out of that dark tunnel three years ago.

Martin told me about the Roses at Glasgow Green. I couldn't make that. Same day as Hands Off Hibs. There were seven thousand rammed inside this tent. When they finished with 'I Am the Resurrection,' Squire's guitar and Mani's bass were so loud he thought they were going to rip the roof right off! It was *religious*. No, *not* religious. *Spiritual. Massive* difference.

It's ironic US Christians are so often right-wing conservatives but the New Testament is a *socialist* manifesto. I've a friend, Rosie, who quoted from the Gospel of Matthew. *According to Jesus, it is easier for a camel to go through the eye of a needle than for a rich man to enter the kingdom of God.* This sentiment is echoed in the Qur'an.

My mind drifts again. I recall Mum returning after collecting for Christian Aid, describing traipsing up and down tenements in Moat or Hutchison where folks always gave her something. But the Polwarth mansions we passed 15 minutes ago, Mercs in the drive? Doors were slammed in her face. Anne gave an ironic chuckle, adding that on her works nights out, she and the other secretaries shoved tenners into the kitty, while the managers would dig pennies from their bulging wallets.

Back in the room, I wonder if that camel and needle touch-stone would include someone winning the Pools? Unlike most of the guys he toiled beside in the tyre factory, Grandad injected colour into his weekly slog by being a voracious reader. But he did share a common vice. Gambling.

Long before bookmaking became legal in 1961, men would keep an eye out for the bookie's runner, exchanging notes for a slip on the corner by the Craigentinny shops. Everyone placing bets on the Musselburgh horse races or Powderhall greyhounds did so under a nom-de-plume. Since Grandad's surname was King, his was Rex. So what if Rex's reverse forecast or *Evening News* 'Spot the Ball' hit the jackpot?

If The Bible's not partitioning God's children between rich and poor, us and them, it's good or bad. How does *that* get measured? Families will be split down the middle. Mum goes to North Merchiston church most Sundays. So she's safe. Dad's an atheist. So he's going downstairs. It's like *Sophie's Choice* but instead of siblings, it's the entire human race. *God's* choice. Sounds like the ultimate definition of madness.

Also, you just have to wonder why God cherrypicked who to share his life messages with. Noah and his sons, Abraham, his wife, Sarah, and daughter Hagar, a *slave girl*. If he could create existence, why not share his message with *everyone*. Wars would have stopped back then, when they were still fought with swords, not atom bombs. Those few billionaires who could eradicate world poverty would have done just that. Billions would have discovered joy. Millions of lives would have been saved. Kurt Vonnegut described the closest humans have come to hearing the voice of God was the sound of silence enveloping the World War 1 battlefields when the armistice began.

Suicide, I murmur. Those three whispered syllables prompt Dr Grant to put his pen down. His eyebrows arch.

That was also turned into a black and white issue by their big book. A sin to take your own life? So desperate people, end of their tether, also have an eternity of damnation to look forward to? That Bible Belt again, with their second amendment giving them the right to bear arms. Stash guns in handbags. America has one of the world's highest homicide rates. Yet there are *more* suicides.

Dr Grant nods. Mark. Without a doubt, you're displaying all the symptoms of another bipolar episode.

Now he points a finger. Asks me to visualise my life as a graph.

For most people, their life graph moves along in waves. Like the Firth of Forth on a summer's day. Here he shifts his fingertip up. Down. Is he trying to hypnotise me? Is that how I'm going to be lured into hospital again? Hypnosis? Maybe not as extreme as being injected with droperidol then shackled inside a straightjacket. But I relax.

If this graph is on a scale of one to ten, Mark, most people will coast between three and seven. The downs and ups of life. *Bereavement*? Here he dips his finger. *A new relationship? Childbirth?* The finger rises.

I've got one, Dr Grant. Scotland getting past the first round of the World Cup this time. His finger soars even more and he grins. But his expression alters.

Bipolar individuals can *soar* way beyond seven, into eight, nine, touching *ten*. If we're back in the Firth of Forth, that's a storm coming in from the North Sea, stirring the waves. Here he points to the ceiling. Or crash down, to two, to one.

Now his gesture sinks towards the carpet tiles, signifying the point I sunk to when my parents were compelled to phone an ambulance.

These might be opposite extremes. But they're part of the same condition.

I gaze at the floor. The bipolar depths. Dr Grant allows the symbolism to sink.

Now I need to speak to your dad. I urge you to consider voluntary admittance before your condition deteriorates to the extent you require to be sectioned again.

56

Morningside Young People

I don't feel as ill as three years ago. I don't feel worthless. There's no paranoia. No delusions about infected blood or hostile neighbours or being denounced by Norman Tebbit. This sense of euphoria is the complete opposite. But this is the crux of being bipolar. The highs are as unnatural as the lows.

Always feeling elated is just as alarming as depression. It's almost *worse* because at least there are giveaway signs someone is feeling down. Mania is depression wearing a clown's painted grin. At the dinner table, in the car, at cinema jaunts, on the phone, I subject Mum, Dad, Anne, and my mates, to manic verbal diarrhoea.

I make sweeping statements about finding God but equate organised religion with Karl Marx's opium. I claim to be writing brilliant works of fiction only to lose the thread of their plots and crush screeds of handwritten papers into the bucket.

After my deranged monologue with Dr Grant in the afternoon, the prognosis was to recommend a period of rehabilitation. So this sunny June evening, around the same time as Genoese bars will be bedecked in tartan, saltires, and joyful singing as the Tartan Army anticipate Scotland's Word Cup opener against Costa Rica tomorrow night, and England fans are brandishing their Union flags like matador capes towards Sardinian riot police, I'm striding towards Ward 1A of the Andrew Duncan Clinic. Dad is carrying my holdall. Maybe he feels some guilt about setting the wheels in motion that have led me into psychiatric care again. When I suffered my first psychotic episode in 1987, I was in no position to question my treatment. I was at such a low point on the bipolar scale that hospitalisation was the only way back. At least I can recognise my folks are only looking out for me. I suppose I might be a bit closer to accepting that failing to recognise my mania is another symptom of it.

We're approached by a nurse, around my age, who introduces herself in a Highland lilt. Andrea. Dad hands over my bag. Follows her toward an office to discuss my care plan. I take the opportunity to stroll down the corridor and take in my temporary home.

I pause by a poster. In the central image, teenagers are enjoying a kickabout with a football in a park. Skimming over the caption I notice the legend YPU. I assume this is a reference to soccer trendies. My fertile imagination conjures Young Partick Uproar, although I'm sure the Thistle mob are North Glasgow Express. Maybe their young team?

Dropping my holdall, I rummage into the side pocket where I jammed a notebook and a pen. Grasping the pen, I find a space on the poster and start scrawling something about uniting against Wallace Mercer. Except my hands are shaking. My first attempt is indecipherable.

I score it out, try again in another corner. But the biro runs out of ink. I'm extolling Scotland's fans to oppose Wallace, one of our country's foremost historical figures.

Stepping back, I realise the poster for this YPU firm now looks defaced as a Sighthill subway. So I seize it from the wall and tear it in two, four, then struggle with eight. My face flushed as I vandalise this notice, I realise Dad is standing there, next to the nurse. He asks me what on earth I'm playing at, but in a resigned manner that implies I've confirmed whatever he's been discussing.

I explain I'm just adding a message, showing solidarity with the YPU, adding a clenched fist gesture somewhere between sepia photos of the International Brigades in Spain and the Judean People's Front in *Monty Python's Life of Brian*. I add he wouldn't get it. I accept most of what the crews get up to is anti-social, to say the least, with some ending up in intensive care for no other reason than supporting a different team. But there's common ground. I mention a neighbour from Briarbank Terrace, Marcus, who'd been to Manchester G-Mex back in March for the Happy Mondays and 808 State. He told me there were Guvnors, Gremlins, Red Army, out their faces. Hugging each other.

Dad and the nurse exchange looks. He's still not clear why I was vandalising a poster.

When does graffiti become vandalism, I counter. When do freedom fighters become terrorists? Political slogans, vandalism? My *graffiti* was about Wallace. *No*. Wallace Mercer. Christ.

The woman explains to Dad how everything will appear confusing and *strange* until I start finding my feet. As for the poster? It's for the Young People's Unit.

Thinking aloud, I muse that this sounds like an amalgamation, an alliance. Various firms uniting under one umbrella to oppose Mercer. To keep the Hibs alive?

In a tone reminiscent of a lecturer explaining quantum physics to an audience of school kids, she smiles and points out the Young People's Unit is an inpatient centre for 12 to 17-year-olds.

After I've said my goodbyes to my father, she'll show me around Ward 1A and I will find everyone, patients and staff, a friendly bunch. Resisting an urge to shake his head at my latest rambling outburst, Dad pats my shoulder. He concludes I've to phone if I need anything. There's a payphone just along the corridor. When I glance that way, I notice a lad prowling the adjoining ward, Ward 1. He's wearing a black Lacoste T-shirt and when he clocks my Fila jacket he glares before about-turning. I accept my impression of youthful unity was misguided. That prick must be Ward 1's top dog and he means to take me on at some point. The notion of squaring up to him gives a jolt of adrenaline.

57

Memories Of Green

Andrea escorts me into the lounge. Two elderly ladies are sipping tea and nibbling biscuits. Should I end up emulating Randle McMurphy and imploring my fellow patients to rebel against authority it won't be for the sake of watching the World Series. It will be over the latest episode of *Murder, She Wrote*.

A tired-looking young mother waves plastic toys at a disinterested baby. A teenage girl in flared jeans stares at the TV. Two South Asian men are hunched over a Scrabble board. A middle-aged guy in a tank-top versus a bearded young man with unkempt hair he keeps running his hand through.

A nurse paces over, grinning at me. He's more smartly dressed than most of his colleagues, none of whom are required to wear any uniform beyond a name badge. Wearing a fetching waistcoat, striped shirt, and matching Paisley pattern tie offset with a silver tie clip, he is also fragrant: I jump to the conclusion his top-end aftershave was a gift from his boyfriend.

Parodying a Bond villain, he adopts a comedic Russian accent: *We've been expecting you, Mister Fleming*. Switching back to Edinburgh he tells me he's Adrian. Adey. My wishes are his command. We shake hands.

Andrea explains Adey will handle the rest of the intros, but she'll be in the office if I need to ask anything. When she exits, Adey claps his hands together, attracting the attention of the other patients: his troops. He tells everyone my name. I gaze around. Blank expressions. Nods. The younger Scrabble player glowers. The elderly women could've been sitting on a number 16 bus. The teenage girl stares, eyelids heavy with meds. I nod at each of them, then follow Adey back down the corridor and into a bedroom containing a single bed, bedside cabinet, wardrobe, and sink.

He sweeps an expansive arm around, like a concierge revealing his hotel's most luxurious suite. Says I can settle in. Consulting his watch, he informs me he'll bring around supper in about 20 minutes. Pots of tea and slices of toast. I nod, hoisting my rucksack onto the bed. He adds I can choose my meals for the following week on menu cards before exiting, leaving me to unpack.

Once my clothes are stacked in the rickety wardrobe, I pop a handful of Maltesers into my mouth, stack the paperbacks by the bed. *The Stories of Raymond Carver. Not Not While The Giro*, by James Kelman. *A Fanatic Heart*, by Edna O'Brien. *The Papers of Tony Veitch*, by William McIlvanney.

Tearing open the fresh 20-pack of Marlboros, I spark five and rest them at corners of the ashtray so they fume like incense sticks. Lighting a sixth, I relish the light-headedness provoked by the first draws.

Thrusting the *Blade Runner* soundtrack into my portable player, I fast-forward to 'Memories of Green.' Lie back on the bed. Shutting my eyes, I picture the scene where Rick Deckard suggests to Rachael a story of an orange spider being devoured by its offspring is not a childhood memory, but an implant. My mind drifts further.

I think of my mate, Gavin. He was in my class at Napier until he dropped out and moved back to Cumbernauld. We keep in touch. By phone. Letters. His favourite writers are Henry Miller, Franz Kafka, and Fyodor Dostoevsky, but he's equally passionate about The Fall, Sonic Youth, and Airdrie FC. He's also a punk poet and supported Little Big Dig at several gigs, with poems such as 'Sniffing Glue' celebrating wilder aspects of his North Lanarkshire teens. In the true spirit of the punk/literature DIY crossover, he self-published several poetry zines.

This Vangelis track, with its serene piano, always reminds me of his piece, 'Hitler's Piano Player.' Whatever Gav's original intention, my soaring imagination has conjured its own scenario.

On the railway platforms at the concentration camps, I picture the SS officers making their arbitrary decisions. Those to be spared because they were fit enough for heavy manual work. Children, elderly, ill or disabled individuals would be sent to the showers. But within that second queue, the Nazis were always on the lookout for artists and musicians. Even sociopathic murderers needed entertainment, so they would recruit members for the camp orchestra or individuals with a talent for portraiture. Seeing this as a last, gasp chance of a reprieve, people would attempt to feign skills.

Prisoners declaring artistic talents would be led into a room where the commandant was seated, waiting patiently. Faced with a blank canvas, a brush, and a palette, anyone claiming to be an artist would have minutes to conjure a likeness. The officer would click his fingers, inspect their work. If this person had produced a decent portrait they'd be led into the hut reserved for privileged prisoners, joining the fortunate ones tasked with sketching sanitised versions of the camp's activities. For propaganda bulletins. If the commandant saw a game but ultimately poor attempt, the prisoner would be marched back to the queue for the showers. In another room, a gleaming piano looted from a Jewish apartment awaited the wishful candidates who'd professed musical aptitude. Again, the commandant would listen for a short while before making his decision.

While events *could* have happened this way, my fertile brain is insisting they *did*. The floating melody is the sound of some brave soul improvising music, perhaps working discordancy into a jazzier element, his life hanging by a thread.

The track concludes. In my daydream, the pianist, whether genuinely accomplished or touching a keyboard for the first time, always constructs this beautiful song. Lives.

I visualise the scene where Deckard holds a photo, supposedly showing Rachael as a child with her mother. As he stares at this image, for a split second, shadows flicker and the scene comes to life. Ridley Scott presents the viewer with the essence of photography: an impression of glancing through a window into history.

I switch off before 'Tales of the Future' kicks in with its more bombastic synths. Fumbling into the side pocket of my holdall, I produce a notebook. While I'm incarcerated, I've got work to do. I remember the psychiatrist doing his rounds of Ward 5 in 1987. How writing short stories was seen as a positive step in my rehabilitation after I'd been sectioned. So I'll be writing my way out of Ward 1A.

Flipping pages, I come across scribbles from the 'Hands Off Hibs' rally. Quotes I obtained in The Clan for the fanzine article I'll finish. Brian's poem is my starting point. But when I review the other scrawls, pretty much the only decent entry. Most of the individuals whose opinions I courted chose not to go into too much detail about what the loss of their beloved football club would mean to them. They opted for poisonous personal attacks on Wallace Mercer. One Hearts supporter suggested a spoof quote from Mrs Mercer. Amongst the squiggles and Pils stains: *never mind the Hobos, imagine having a fucking walrus on top of you every time the fucking Viagra kicks in...*

Grasping the Carver anthology, I flick onto the first story. 'Fat.' It describes an obese man being served in a diner, the waitress fascinated by his 'long, thick, creamy fingers.' Placing the paperback down, I gaze at my own quivering digits. I recall how I kept staring at my hands the first time I dropped magic mushrooms as if, after 20-odd years, I was only just taking in the marvels of biology. But I clock the ochre discolouration around the fingertips where I hold my cigarettes. I think of Mum noting the tainted skin, telling me it put her in mind of her dad and his protracted death by emphysema.

I focus on Vangelis, 'The Tao of Love,' with its Far Eastern chimes and washes of synthesiser. Springing up, I jack-knife the fag into the ashtray, extinguishing the others. I've decided I want a proper introduction to each of my ward mates.

When I exit my room I bump into a female nurse with short peroxide spikes. Ali, I say, reading her badge. She smiles, introducing herself with a handshake. After referring to myself as Ward 1A's latest inmate, to which she chuckles, I go on to compliment her hair, informing her she reminds me of Honey Bane. When she shrugs at this, I add that Honey fronted the Fatal Microbes, creating a further layer of incomprehension. I explain they were a punk band, and Honey went on to enjoy a solo career, including the first single issued on the Crass label, the 'You Can Be You' EP, released when she was a 15-year-old runaway. Crass, as in Anarchy, Peace and Freedom. Banned from the Roxy. Punk is Dead. This tirade of gibberish baffles her.

Ali admits defeat: she was a bit young for punk. Did Fatal Microbes or Crass have many hits? I scoff at the notion of Crass topping the charts, recalling the Merchiston Youth Club – the Merky – where we hung around as teenagers and were allowed to take our own records. Once I handed Crass's

'Shaved Women' to the DJ, an upbeat number sung by Eve Libertine. Anticipating the moment the DJ would play two or three punk singles that would clear the dancefloor after the wall-to-wall disco and Northern Soul the majority of the punters danced to, inciting a dozen youths to draw everyone's attention for anarchic minutes, I nipped to the loo.

There I got into an altercation with a pissed lad I recognised from a Tynie remedial class. He claimed I'd given him a funny look and I was fucking dead before falling backwards and whacking his head off the sink. When I went to help him up he pushed me away, insisted he just wanted to sit there. I could smell the Evo-Stik on his breath.

Returning to the main hall, I discovered the DJ had stuck on the wrong side. You could pogo to 'Shaved Women.' 'Reality Asylum,' a six-minute spoken word rant, demanded to be listened to, not danced to, its excoriating irreligious sentiment resembling the bile frothing from 12-year-old Regan in *The Exorcist*. I heard *Jesu. Cock fear. Cunt fear. Woman fear*. Segueing into *warfare*. Gaping at the empty dancefloor and baffled faces, as Eve Libertine concluded about Jesus dying for his own sins, *not mine*, I visualised a tumbleweed trundling over the floorboards.

I explain Crass were more an albums band. Well. More an albums and vegetarian communes band. As for Honey, she went on to appear on *Top of the Pops* in 1981.

Ali enquires what modern bands I listen to, and I wax lyrical about Madchester, and how The Stone Roses debut album is the greatest music I've heard since the heyday of punk 13 years before. She informs me there's a lad I'll have to meet in the next ward, Stevie who's also a massive fan. Glancing at her watch, she bids me farewell, concluding by saying she'll ask her older brother about Crash.

Another nurse walks past, tall and leggy, with dark skin and shoulder-length hair. She halts, gives me a wondrous smile, and introduces herself as Sunita. When I ask where her accent is from, she tells me she was born in Jaffna in Sri Lanka. Like a sizeable percentage of twentysomethings from Britain, I have no clue about the country's former colonies, and when I ask if Sri Lanka is bigger than Skye, she tells me it's nearer the size of Scotland.

Moving on from my ignorance of the former Empire's geography, I tell her I like what I've seen of Ward 1A so far. I go on to mention my experiences of the IPCU in 1987, where nurses often prised patients apart, like ice hockey umpires. Although I only ever witnessed this on a couple of occasions, my manic train of thought is overblowing these skirmishes.

An imposing man with blond hair, wearing a pale blue suit, strolls by. Waving at Sunita, he heads into the office. Dr Maher, she tells me. When I announce he was separated at birth from Christopher Biggins, she glares for conjuring a vision she'll now have to suppress whenever their paths cross.

58

Black And

Ward 1A of the Royal Edinburgh Hospital has been my temporary home for almost 45 minutes and I'm already restless. Flicking through the Carver compilation, I thumb to the shortest story, 'Popular Mechanics,' describing a domestic crisis in one and a half pages. I've read this so many times the nightmarish scene is ingrained.

Checking my cigarettes, there are seven left from the 20-pack I bought after asking Dad to stop off by Irvine's on Cowan Road on the way here. I pluck another out. Decide not to spark it. Chainsmoking to the point of running out when I've no idea who I can cadge off will make me even more fidgety.

When I worked in the Scottish Record Office a few months ago, if I ran out of fags I knew who I could tap. I'd a network of fellow smokers to pester, whether that was the other casual assistants, the reps who delivered archive Sasine documents to the customers, or punters in the Penny Black around the corner. I think of the latter.

One of the other regulars was a lad I knew as Figsy, another veteran of the Edinburgh punk scene. Until I'd a couple of pints under my belt I was wary of approaching him. He earned a reputation for being a nutjob.

Back in the late 1970s, when the battle lines between youth cults were drawn up around musical tastes and fashion sense, there was one notorious Saturday when gangs of punks and mods arranged a set-to in the city centre. This was an escalation of incidents the night before at the Merky, when brawls erupted between mods from Tollcross and Oxgangs, and punks from Gorgie and Shandon. At one point, Pauline, the singer of my band, The Seduced, was beaten up.

Princes Street shoppers found themselves immersed in a variation of *Quadrophenia*, mobs wearing parkas or biker jackets fighting running battles. I recall Figsy wielding a bicycle chain like a demented gladiator, chasing a bunch of terrified mods through Boots.

Later that rowdy afternoon, strolling through Princes Street Gardens with a couple of other punks, we spotted 50 or so mods hanging around the Ross Bandstand. One of the lads, a guy with a striped black and gold barnet named Devlin, punched the air. Began hollering the Angelic Upstarts chorus: *I'm an upstart, hey! Whatcha gonna do? I'm an upstart, listen! I'm talking to you!* The three of us legged it up to Princes Street, a stampede of two-tone shoes inspiring our tactical retreat.

The Penny Black sometimes seemed to be a haven for drinkers with a violent past. One of the others I could count on for smokes was Tony, a mate of Keith, the Hibs Boy that Alex, John, Splodge and I worked beside. Tony would describe the formative Casual era, long before the CCS fell under the police radar and their train departure times were printed alongside the details for official Hibs buses on the *Evening News* back page. Hair-raising tales of pincer movement ambushes on the wasteground by the Playhouse when Aberdeen were down or Motherwell or the Old Firm were through. Weekend breaks to Millwall.

Tony came to my rescue last year after I bought the *Blackadder The Third* box-set for Dad's Christmas, then got so guttered at the office reps' party I left the videos in the pub before exiting in a stupor. He came chasing after me, thrusting the bag into my grasp as I was falling aboard a number 44 in St Andrew Square.

Not only was I pestering workmates for snouts, I was also tapping them for money. As a temp, I was paid weekly, rather than the salary my full-time colleagues received. Fridays, I cashed my £90 giro in the Post Office on Waterloo Place, a chunk dissipating as I repaid these short-term loans.

The temptation is too much. Lighting up, I stretch back on the bed, exhaling towards the tiles. I dwell on the turn of events that have brought me here. Revisiting that butterfly effect notion, that the chemical imbalances that came to a head, or more fittingly, sunk to a depth, three years ago, were instigated by the trauma of adolescent abuse. In Dr Grant's words, mental injury, rather than illness. Life is full of chance moments that can pitch you off in a different direction. Coincidences.

I think of two of the most stunning examples of the latter. Aged 19, during my first long-term relationship with Louise, I often stayed over. On the wall of the spare bedroom in her folks' Newington home, there was a painting, like an illustration from a nursery rhyme, of a sledge being pulled through snow by a hare, its passengers two fairies. The same painting hung in the janitor's office in my primary school. If Mrs Marwick sent me to the janitor when I was feeling sick, I'd perch on a chair, feet dangling, sipping a glass of warm milk. I knew every inch of that fantastical scene.

A few weeks before Christmas 1983, I went out with a girl I met in the Hooch. Diane. One of her best friends was Petra, daughter of the politician Margo MacDonald, a stalwart of Scotland's right to self-determination, and campaigner for tolerance zones for Edinburgh prostitutes. Petra went on to marry Charlie Reid of The Proclaimers. I first heard of Charlie and his twin Craig when they played in a punk band, Black Flag, and practised alongside The Axidents in the Blair Street catacombs, where the Reid brothers were known as 'the skinhead Buddy Hollys.'

Diane's dad once got tickets for Hector Nicol at the Telecomms Club on Gorgie Road, but couldn't make it. She asked if I fancied going, unsure if someone who played in a 'cool' alternative band would be interested in music hall comedy. I was over the moon.

Paisley-born Nicol was a bawdy comedian and singer, a veteran of social clubs and smokers. While his observations of working-class Scottish life were an obvious influence on Billy Connolly, his material was way too blue for TV. But his was also a classic tears of a clown story, with family tragedies almost prompting premature retirement. Two of his three sons died in harrowing circumstances, one choking while eating, another fatally stabbed by a stranger at an Edinburgh bus stop when he was 19, the perpetrator of his motiveless murder only 15. Nicol decided to focus on his idiosyncratic and hilarious stage routines, channelling his darker experiences into serious roles in *Just A Boy's Game* and *A Sense of Freedom*. My mate, Grum was also a huge fan of his comic persona, and having loaned me a couple of his albums we could imitate many of his routines word-for-word.

Living in Carrick Knowe, five minutes from the club, Diane suggested I pick her up. She gave me her address. I remembered Mum and Dad's first home in Edinburgh was in this neck of the woods. I ran her house number by Dad. It was the same house.

I once asked Dad about his first impressions of Scotland. He said the biggest hurdle was the accent. A neighbour came to that door and announced: *yir lum's up!* Asking him to repeat this didn't help. Then the guy hauled him out to the street and pointed at smoke pluming from the chimney. Dad phoned for the fire brigade: the first of only two times my parents were forced to dial 999.

Stubbing out the fag, I decide to explore. I spot a figure coming out of Ward 1. When our eyes meet my heart soars. Coincidences? I hurry towards him and grasp his hand. This psychiatric nurse is Ian, my best mate at Craiglockhart primary.

In the moments we shake hands, a montage of memories floods. The smell of glue from building Airfix warplanes. Swapping football cards from bubblegum packets. Comparing the Apollo 1969 medals his Dad picked up at Shell garages with the Mexico World Cup 1970 souvenirs Dad collected when he bought Esso petrol from Willie Woodburn's garage at Longstone – a former Rangers centre-half and the last British player to receive a life ban for his disciplinary record. Going to see *Goldfinger* then replaying the Oddjob scene with a Dairylea Triangle lid. Cutting Napoleonic dragoons from Corn Flakes packets. We went on to the same secondary but hadn't shared any classes. By the end of First Year our friendship had waned to chance meetings in the playground. Fifteen years later, we're reunited by fate.

I regurgitate long-forgotten stories. One time he told me his eldest sister was with her boyfriend in the queue outside The Americana, Edinburgh's first 'discotheque,' when one of the Tollcross Rebels, the local street gang, who wore *Clockwork Orange* gear, told this boyfriend his shoulder-length hair made him look like a *poof*. The boyfriend nutted him, his bowler hat rolling into traffic.

He admits no memory of this. So I fast-forward, reminding him of the Stranglers badges he wore in our English class: a white one printed with 'Black And,' and a black badge with 'And White.'

He asks why I'm here, but when I mumble *depression* it seems as inadequate as describing photosynthesis as 'flowers shagging.'

59

No X-Mas For Junkies

I sit by the table where the two Asian guys are intent on Scrabble. I think of Dad's former boss, Liston, his chief drinking partner now they're both retired. He served in the Army in India and has taught Dad a few Urdu phrases which he now uses every time he collects the Sunday papers from the Pakistani newsagents. Phonetically, one sounded like *Bo Tunder, Hai*. I'm sure this translated as: *Sunny day*.

I try this on the older gent. *Bo Tunder, Hai?* He frowns, asking me to repeat myself. It's Urdu, I insist. He informs me he's a Hindi speaker.

I ask his name. Prakash, he replies. I announce I'm the new kid on the block, from Shandon. Not too far away. A civil servant. I like writing. I used to play guitar in a band. My favourite group? The Stone Roses. Overall, Sex Pistols. The Clash. And The Fall. Everyone has a shortlist but who can ever put them in order? He squints as if I'm still mangling Urdu. Favourite films? Blade Runner. Some Like It Hot. I ask Prakash to tell me about himself, suggesting he imagines I'm Eamonn Andrews and I've sprung my famous red book on him.

He was a train driver in India. His family emigrated to Uganda but when Idi Amin expelled the tens of thousands of Asian settlers in 1972 they moved to Leith. He worked in Central Station.

I let him know about my former band, Little Big Dig. We practised in Leith and managed to get into that station four years before. It was boarded up but you could squeeze through a gap in the fencing. It was weird being inside this vast, derelict station. Rubbish everywhere. Rainwater leaking from dozens of shattered panes above the rusting gantries where swarms of pigeons flapped.

We took lots of photos, including the ticket office. He smiles. That was where he worked. He thought the trains were ugly compared to the steam engines he drove. Favourite films? One was *North West Frontier*, about the sectarian strife during The Raj. Part of it was filmed in Rajasthan, his childhood home.

I switch my attention to the younger lad and introduce myself. Nodding, he plucks one of his letters, gazing at it, pops it back. Then he glares, running his other hand through his wild curls. Tells me he's Jansher, from Liberton. Studying Astronomy at Heriot-Watt.

Prakash elaborates Jansher's family are from Pabna, and he is a Bengali. Jansher scratches at his locks, stares at both of us for a while, murmuring, *Bangladesh*. Sighing, he shifts in his chair, returning his attention to the Scrabble.

Leaving the table, I locate a spare chair between the young woman offering toys to her child and the teenage girl. I prise out of the teenager her name is Tanya, from Saughton Mains. She's on the ward until a space becomes available at the YPU. But she fixates on the wildlife documentary on TV.

Switching my attention to the older woman, I ask her baby's name. Clara. She's Chrissie. I tell her she sounds like she could star in *Last of The Summer Wine*. She's from Halifax. All I know about Halifax is their local team are Halifax Town, and from childhood Subbuteo charts I recall they played in blue with tangerine trimmings. Light blue and white stripes last season, she informs me, like Argentina. *Wish they played like bloomin' Argentina*, she adds.

I laugh about Argentina losing their opening game at *Italia 90*, 1-0 to Cameroon. She also tells me Town's nickname. The Shaymen. I say my cousin Ross's best buddy Colin plays in The Shamen. She asks which position? Vocals, guitar, and keyboards.

I pace out of the lounge, back to my room. Sparking up a Marlboro I check out the view. I think of Basil Fawlty countering a cantankerous guest's complaint about her room's view by apologising for the lack of wildebeests. Ward 1A is on the ground floor so my vista will be the car park. Closing the curtains, I eject the Vangelis cassette, replacing it with Killing Joke's debut album. When 'The Wait' starts pulsating into the room I take lingering draws, studying myself in the mirror above the sink.

I don't think I've changed that much since I saw them with Boots for Dancing at Heriot-Watt Student Union 10 years ago. Punk bands were barred from that venue, but Killing Joke were booked after denying they fell into this cliched category. Instead of spiked hair, it's stepped: long on top, razored around the sides. Running both taps. I fill the sink. Dunk my head in. I step back, water soaking my T-shirt, running my fingers through the strands so the hair looks gelled. Nodding to Geordie's crunching guitar, I stab the dowt into the ashtray.

I stride back to the lounge. Prakash is in an armchair, intent on an *Evening News*. Janser is mesmerised by lionesses stalking zebras in the Serengeti Plain. The two older women have commandeered the Scrabble board. I make a beeline for them. One has white curls, reminiscent of Harpo Marx. She gives me a beaming smile. When I introduce myself, she replies her name is Victoria.

Her companion has dark hair, pinched features, and glares over her spectacles. She is Kathleen and has a good word, if I don't mind. Victoria rises, gives an exaggerated yawn, then releases a resounding fart before sitting back down. Catching her mischievous expression, I burst out laughing. Tears well as I watch Kathleen jotting her score for 'Quizzical.'

Victoria farts again. Kathleen slams down her pencil and drags her chair away from the table, the impact of her petulant withdrawal diffused by the time it takes. Glaring at us both, she shuffles over to sit before the TV.

After Victoria departs, I tip all the letters into the board, shuffling them. Thinking of those speed chess tournaments where a grandmaster faces multiple opponents, I begin snatching letters. My theme takes its inspiration from two of my main cultural obsessions – the lyrics of Mark E. Smith and the words of Glaswegian writer James Kelman.

I place NO XMAS FOR JUNKIES across the middle, paraphrasing 'No X-mas for John Quays', the climactic track on The Fall's debut album. I incorporate the final S into PSY-CHOMAFIA, from their first single's B-side. Then, references to the flipside of Festival City: AIDS. HIV. Although I doubt it's suggested in the rules, consonants are perfect for gang acronyms. CCS. YLT. MCF. GJ. I add schemes. NIDDRIE, MOREDUN. INCH. GRANTON. Kelman is name-checked with NOTNOTGIRO. I complete the board in minutes with few letters omitted. Here's the cover for my debut short story anthology.

60

Adored

My cigarettes are burning like joss-sticks when there's a knock at the door. A lad hovers, wearing a Burberry shirt and baggy jeans, with a lank ginger bowl-cut. He clutches a Coda bag rammed with cassettes. Scuffing in, he offers a limp handshake. Introduces himself as Stevie. Says he's heard I'm a big Roses fan. When I give him a thumbs-up, he plucks a cassette from his stash. I see the iconic John Squire action painting.

I feed the tape into my player and when Mani's towering bassline introduces 'I Wanna Be Adored,' I offer a Marlboro. When we're sparked, I ask what other cassettes he has. He tips the bag over my bed. Inspiral Carpets. Charlatans. Happy Mondays. Northside. Mock Turtles. The Farm.

It was his birthday yesterday. 19. When I was that age I was into Killing Joke. Fire Engines. The Fall. Siouxsie and the Banshees. He's heard of Siouxsie and the Banshees. We chat about music. A common denominator. During 'Waterfall' he glances sideways. Asks why I'm here.

I explain the bipolar diagnosis. How my meds are being upped because I've been getting so manic. How I struggle to sleep. Last night I ended up prowling the corridors, noising up the night nurses.

Stevie describes his own situation. Mouth running on overdrive. Chewing gum as if it's burning his tongue. He's from Clermiston. Was running with the local gang. Young Clerrie Derry in his old man's day. Now they're CSF. Hearts Boys. Because he was one of the tallest cunts, he was ayeways ordered to the front before they steamed in.

Takes an urgent drag, gawking at his trainers. Reliving painful memories in every sense.

Sniggering, I butt in. Ordered to the front, eh? The taller cunts and the bams. Going toe to toe with Hibs or Aberdeen, you'd be the cannon fodder. Like the Scottish soldiers on the Empire's battlefields!

The fucking Hibees? There were just as many of them around Clerrie. He was an obvious target. Spent half his fucking puff pure getting jumped. Outside chippies. In the Clerrie Inn or The Rainbow. Told by Hibees if he was ever spotted further east than the Wimpy in Prinny, he'd get fucking banjoed. A six-foot-tall Clerrie cunt with this hair could be pure clocked a block away. A fucking walking red rag. Red man walking.

Here his description of pervasive violence prompts a giggling fit dissolving into an alarming coughing spree.

They were ayeways outnumbered cause the Hibs attracted lads from *everywhere*. Any part of the town. Midlothian. East and West Lothian. Even gadges who followed Hearts or the Huns. But the CSF were into the same nonsense as the Huns. Union Jacks and red hands at Tynie. He escaped the aggro by raving and the Madchester bands. Dropping ectoes every weekend. Pure tipped him over the fucking edge. The dance scene got him away from the kickings, but the comedowns were fucking brutal. This went on for months, till he just couldn't take it. Pretty much locked himself away in his bedroom.

I tell him *snap*. Apart from the hooligan stuff. Couldn't say when I was last in a fight, apart from swinging drunken punches at mods at the Merky youth club. Last time I decked someone in genuine anger was when another boy tried to steal my wee sister's tricycle. Mind you, his oldest brother was in Gorgie Jungle. Had to keep a low profile after that!

*

At 9 p.m. we queue for our meds. Marvelling at the dose of tablets Kathleen and Victoria are issued, I tell Victoria they must sound like human maracas. Grinning, she fires her customary riposte.

After necking my chlorpromazine I settle into the armchair. On the news, Nelson Mandela is addressing crowds during his tour of the USA. He gazes over a sea of humanity, features beaming. The newscaster contrasts this with the view imposed on him by the apartheid regime: four walls of a four-metre-squared cell for 27 years. Martyn Lewis mentions the title bestowed on him by his white supremacist captors: prisoner 466/64.

A film starts. *Amityville Horror*. I've read the book, based on a 'true' story about a Dutch colonial house on Long Island. A young couple, George and Kathy Lutz and their three kids, move into the house a year after a 23-year-old, Ronald DeFeo Jnr murdered his parents, two sisters and two brothers there with a rifle. The Lutz family are exposed to inexplicable phenomena, leading them to believe the house is possessed. I decide I'll get more engrossed if I kill the lights, so I flick them off.

Margot Kidder and James Brolin play the newlyweds, while Rod Steiger overacts his role as a priest. I abandon the conflict between good and evil when I feel my meds kicking in.

In the corridor, I gaze over to Ward 1 and spot their Top Boy. I decide to take the piss. Thinking of Basil Fawlty again, I goose-step towards him. He turns away before noticing. So I skulk into the toilets. Now I imagine I'm in some propaganda film produced by leftists during the Third Reich. Instead of Hollywood's melodramatic paranormality, I think of the genuine terror of Jewish families on Kristallnacht, the men in swastika armbands selecting which houses to order the residents out into the street for beatings. Pressing my ear against the cubicle door, I knock and knock. But I'm startled when one of the night nurses shines a torch into my face.

*

On the table sits a stack of blank menu cards. I decide to complete all of them, ticking boxes at random, recalling names to scribble at the foot. I'm sure mealtimes will be a pleasant surprise.

Heading back to my room for a smoke, I pass the empty office. Notice a planner above the desk, the vagaries of shifts, meetings, training sessions, admissions, and appointments indicated by different colour codes and symbols. But I see an abstract design and spend five minutes re-arranging the arrows and blocks.

*

In the TV lounge, I'm experiencing the eternal curse of the Scotland football fan: World Cup disaster déjà vu. Our fifth consecutive tournament but we're losing to Costa Rica. Richard Gough limped off just after half-time, then three minutes later the Central Americans scored.

I'm mesmerised by the way I can anticipate the direction each pass is going to take. Becoming immersed in the game's flow is hypnotic. I visualise Andy Roxburgh's pre-match diagrams. Emphatic arrows for the ideal box-to-box moves. The fluid symmetry of Alex McLeish and Roy Aiken finding Jim Bett and Paul McStay. But when Maurice Malpas has all the time in the world to cross towards Mo Johnston only to get caught in possession, I realise nobody could predict what this lot might do next.

61

Psych Ward Breakout

Ward 1A is an open ward, so there's a degree of flexibility about visiting. If family offer to escort the patient somewhere different to chill, this is seen as a valuable aspect of rehabilitation.

Dad drives to Holyrood Park, heading up the winding road to pull in by Dunsapie Loch. Tossing bread scraps toward mallards, mute swans, coots, and black-headed gulls instigates a feeding frenzy.

Feeling a similar craving, I spark a Marlboro. Inhale the smoke to every pore of my lungs while the folks are intent on *The Scotsman* crossword. When they're not looking, I thumb another from the packet, lighting it from the previous one.

Grinding out the dowt, I ease into the passenger seat. The newspaper is folded away and we make for Morningside. When we stop at the lights by the Commonwealth Pool I spot two guys I used to work beside in the Scottish Widows. I know they'll have been to Braidwoods, the pub on West Preston

Street where we spent two-hour lunch breaks engrossed in videos like *Kentucky Fried Movie*, *The Thing*, and *Friday the 13th* on the large screen. Eight or so years ago seems a lifetime.

*

When I wave my goodbyes and stroll back into the ward, Ali heads toward me. She explains I can't go into my bedroom. Decorators are giving the rooms a lick of paint.

But I decide to grab the Raymond Carver paperback. Dust sheets cover the floor and two guys in white overalls are touching up the window sills. The older one tells me I shouldn't be in here, the walls are still wet. His mate reminds me of somebody. I ask his name and when he says Ally Stevenson, the penny drops. His brother, Bobby is the convener of the Union Jack bus. But this painter tells me he's a Jambo with no time for Bobby's weegie allegiances.

Pacing into the middle of the room I peer into the mirror above the sink. There's a white streak down the sleeve of my black Next T-shirt. I shrug. Spying a large pot of emulsion, I extract a brush from a jar of water. Digging it into the paint, I draw a stripe on the other arm to match the stain, then paint bold stripes across my chest.

Laughing, Ally asks if I'm creating a St Mirren strip, says he hates those bastards for lying down to the Tims so they'd win the league four years ago. Would've been their first title since 1960, the year he was born. But I point out his own team just needed one point. The night after Albert Kidd had broken thousands of hearts at Dens Park, my mates and I ended up in Cat's Pyjamas. Abbeyhill. Closest nightclub to Easter Road. Skirmishes between losers and gloaters kept erupting. On the dancefloor. At the bar. Around the tables. In the cloakroom queue. In the bogs. The bouncers must have ejected 50% of the punters who paid at the door, teeing up more punch-ups in Abbeyhill.

Studying my handiwork in the mirror, I drag the bristles across my face, Adam Ant-style. The painters glance at each other. I'm sure they could write a book about the behaviour they've witnessed while decorating the Royal Ed.

I've decided to invoke the warrior spirit behind 'Kings of the Wild Frontier,' visualising the Ants at Valentino's in 1980, the twin-Burundi drumbeat thundering. Minutes later I'm jogging up Tipperlin Road, intending to look up my mate, Silly. He lives with his parents in an Ashley Terrace tenement.

When I arrive at his stair, the main door is open. I duck inside, sweat dripping as I climb the two flights. When he answers his front door he looks shocked. He tells me he'll put the kettle on. We can watch the New Order video he bought at the weekend. Relaxing in an armchair, fag already lit, I hear him on the telephone. Ten minutes later the buzzer goes. He tramps along the hallway, speaking into the entryphone. *Hello, Allen. I'll tell him you're here.*

Silly reappears. I glower and demand to know why he grassed me up? He reminds me I'm still an inpatient. That's why my dad is waiting in the car to take me back where I need to be to get better. When I see him attempting to keep a straight face, my expression mellows. I tell him this isn't the first time I've made a James Hunt of myself today. He studies my warpaint. Nowhere near, he suggests, winking.

62

Birthday

July 1990

I had unexpected visitors yesterday. Alex. Grum. John, lurid crescent scar drawing stares. John's mate, Neil, designated driver. Almost as if they were springing me from incarceration, they marched into Ward 1A, sweeping me up in a flurry of excitable banter, before we squeezed into Neil's car for an exhilarating hurtle across south Edinburgh. I reckon this show of solidarity was partly inspired by a visit to John's I organised after he was discharged from St John's in May, a bunch of us arriving on his doorstep for moral support. What mates do.

Exhaling, I watch the smoke dissipating. Beyond, the breakers crashing over Coldingham Bay have attracted surfers. Serious exponents with wetsuits and boards. Others, like we used to be, content to thrash around with lilos, only T-shirts, football tops or skin to screen us from the icy North Sea.

Mum and Dad picked me up mid-morning and we drove down to St Abbs for a pub lunch at The Haven hotel. Also the venue for numerous sessions over the summers. Depending on the owner at the time, sometimes with lock-ins.

I wolfed a baked potato crammed with succulent fresh prawns smothered in Mary Rose sauce, overloaded with chips. Mum had a crab and lobster salad, recently trapped in local creels. Dad, fresh mackerel pâté.

While I finish my fag, the folks stroll ahead. The sun is splitting gossamer clouds above the small knowe overlooking the beach, Homeli Knoll, christened Pudding Hill by someone in the company a long time ago. A wry smile. My cousin Ross, our mate, Jol and me spent long summer afternoons playing on the rocks surrounding that hillock, reimagining a Stone Age village like Skara Brae in the Orkneys - older than Stonehenge or the Pyramids. Building mammoth traps by draping dried grass over fissures, we were always wary of sabre-toothed tigers or cave bears, although we were too young to introduce anyone wearing fur-bikinis like Loana from *One Million Years B.C.* into our fantasy world.

In later years, we came across a tyre amongst jetsam washed on the rocks, hauled it to the top of Pudding Hill, then released it, envisaging it careering into the sea. Striking an outcrop, it switched direction and hurtled towards the beach, smashing into a windbreak. Instead of pretend carnivores, a posse of irate adults raced in our direction. We took to our heels.

I would've been 16 the last time I felt the exhilaration of catching a wave, hurtling towards the shore, fingers white-knuckled around my lilo's rope grips, fearing being pitched overboard by the savage undertow to gulp briny seawater.

Today is my birthday. 28.

63

Scotland 1 Yugoslavia 1

December 1992

Tomorrow is the office Christmas party. Celebrating the birth of humankind's saviour, binge drinking will commence long before 10 a.m. I'm getting myself in the party mood. Slumped in the settee, I drain another Pils, reach for the last Marlboro. Anne is out with friends so I've got the flat to myself, alternating between Laurel and Hardy videos, and Nirvana's *Nevermind* at increasing volume.

A TV news item catches my eye. Muting the Hi-Fi, I turn up the volume. Slobodan Milosevic has been re-elected president of Serbia. Addressing a rapt audience in Belgrade he seems an unremarkable fiftysomething in a suit. He could be one of the Senior Executive Officers at work.

The podium is draped in red, blue, and white tricolours, some emblazoned with a double-headed white eagle, others the old Yugoslav red star. The camera pans the fervent crowd. Finds a tall Orthodox priest, Karl Marx beard but a polar opposite mindset. Reacting to this leader's words as if he is a Messiah. With different banners, this could be Nuremberg in the 1930s.

Mum used to host foreign language students when Anne and I were still in primary. Their presence in the house was exotic. There was a French girl, Kristianne, who caused a sensation when she joined us during our annual holiday and splashed around in the North Sea wearing the skimpiest two-piece bikini any onlookers had ever set eyes on: way more St Tropez than St Abbs.

There was, Gokce, from Turkey. When his local team, Bursaspor played Dundee United in the Cup Winners Cup, he travelled up to Tannadice, met the squad, and brought back souvenirs, including a satchel bearing the Terrors' badge. Mum sewed tartan over this so I could take it to school.

Another was Pantelis, a portly, jovial Greek, with a jet black beard. He took me to Murrayfield for a Scotland Ireland rugby match which bored me to tears. But also treated me to my only outing to Easter Road's main stand. When I missed who scored a scrambled goal against Dunfermline, he tapped the shoulder of the man in front, who asked him if he was French. That season Rangers won their first title since 1964, a point secured at Easter Road the following March preventing Celtic's 10th successive championship. I remember being aghast at the news footage. The 38,500 fans seemed to be all bluenoses. But Hibs were runners-up, four points above Celtic. In September we beat Liverpool at home in the UEFA Cup, although the English team won on aggregate, progressing to lift the trophy.

The summer before I started secondary, Pantelis and I were absorbed by the World Cup in West Germany. With Famous Five veteran Willie Ormond at the helm, Scotland had qualified for the first time since 1958. Greece hadn't, so he was supporting his neighbours, Yugoslavia. They were in our group, instigating a jocular rivalry as we were glued to the TV. Our match was drawn 1-1, a left-footed strike by Joe Jordan equalising what had been the only goal scored against us during the tournament. But when news filtered through of Brazil's 3-0 victory over Zaire, making their goal difference one better than us, the Yugoslav fans celebrated reaching the next round. They'd hammered the Africans 9-0.

Yugoslavia finished bottom of their 2nd round group, losing to West Germany, Poland, and Sweden. The highlight of the remainder of the tournament was watching Holland's 'total football.' Spearheaded by Johan Cruyff's mercurial skills, they defeated holders Brazil in the semi-final. The Dutch finished runners-up to the West German hosts.

Did any of those supporters anticipate the barbaric implosion of their nation within their lifetimes? Yugoslavia is sinking into an ultra-nationalistic morass, stoked by right-wing politicians like this besuited rabble-rouser, hankering for a medieval notion of a Greater Serbia. Endorsed by the once multi-ethnic Yugoslav National Army and Red Star Belgrade hooligans who now have guns.

Disgusted by the murderous fervour in so many eyes, I switch off.

*

Flicking through my address book, I stop at random. *Lisa. Reflections.* An attractive 21-year-old hairdresser, blonde bob razored into an extreme step. This had been the epitome of chic in 1985, but Alex referred to her as 'Bully Beef,' the *Beano* character with a pudding bowl crop.

According to rumours, Reflections' owners paid protection to Southeast Edinburgh gangsters. The night I met Lisa coincided with heavies turning up to demand outstanding donations. As we slow-danced to Madonna's 'Crazy For You,' we could hear a blunt instrument crashing against the locked doors.

Violence seemed to be stalking us. The journey to Lisa's at Gracemount on the night bus was undertaken against a backdrop of aggressive choirs upstairs, howling respective Hibs and Celtic anthems. As the rowdy banter escalated into goading, the fuse was sparked by someone roaring *CCS!* A mass brawl erupted along the ceiling, as if we were snogging below a rodeo. The driver stopped while awaiting the response to his 999 call.

Reminiscing about that wild night would be an ice-breaker before asking her out. So I dial her number, slugging from a half-pint tumbler containing the remaining alcohol I could find: Rosé.

When the phone answers, I don't recognise the voice. I ask for Lisa. The woman informs me her daughter is at a hen party. When I ask, whose, she answers, *hers*. Mumbling about passing on my congratulations, I hang up. I'm already focused on the next old flame for rekindling. Wendy, a Prestonpans goth I met in Cat's Pyjamas on Albert Kidd day. After dialling her number, I cringe at the unobtainable monotone.

Lifting the wine from the table, I seek refuge with Kurt Cobain.

64

Ice Cold In Edinburgh

Staring towards the Banana Flats, I recall that short-lived bid for freedom when I stormed out the hospital, dripping in paint. One in a long line of manic episodes. It's been two years since I was discharged, exiting the ward with the good wishes of the staff rather than instigating a frantic search party.

It seems hard to reconcile then and now. Months of insomnia and paranoia. Self-harming leading to Mum's desperate 999 call. Sectioning. Three years of relative wellbeing. The onset of manic behaviour. Mania. Glee. Insomnia. Excessive drinking. Promiscuity. An embarrassing flirtation with boorish right-wing politics. Hospitalisation again. It's all so detached from the person I've become, I can look back with an embarrassed smile. As opposed to the nightmares Mum and Dad will always experience.

Arresting my attention from the paperwork cluttering my desk, I observe the sprawling flats. The staff on this floor often receive voyeuristic distractions from our tasks. There's a lad who spends much of his day freaking out to hard house. Carving shapes. Waving lightsticks. Blowing into a whistle. Two weeks ago, someone at the top level clambered out of a window and spent 20 minutes clinging to a ledge until a fire engine arrived. Everyone is wary of two particular flats: one where eggs were launched at Eli, a Brazilian-born finance manager whose skin tone elicited shouts of *paki bastard*; another where someone pockmarked the office with an air rifle.

My phone goes. It's Bill, the office receptionist, an ex-lighthousekeeper whose Santa-like beard belies an expletive-peppered Leith accent. He grew up near Cables Wynd and often fascinates me with childhood stories. Watching the wrestling in the State Cinema on Great Junction Street, the pugilists firing themselves up in the pub over the road while awaiting their summons to the ring. Playing in the scrapyard on the site where those flats now loom, where he once discovered World War 1 French bayonets long as swords. Today's excitement is that a sales rep dropped by, leaving a Christmas pressie. When I enquire which rep, he replies the dirty blonde that wants to suck your fucking balls dry, before chortling and hanging up.

After retrieving the package, I tear it open. A case of four bottles of Spanish Rioja. I read the note.

Dear Mark. Have a great Christmas and a fab New Year. All the best to you. Thanks for all your custom! Look forward to keeping you supplied with quality stationery in 1993! Lynda x

As a Scottish Office administrative assistant, my job description involves everything from ordering sundry office equipment, photocopy paper to marker pens, to testing the fire alarms each Tuesday morning. But today's priority was booking a flotilla of taxis for Cupid's on Waterloo Place. In time-honoured tradition, a turkey meal will precede the disco, where Slade, Wizzard, and the other usual suspects will provide the soundtrack to almost 100 office clerks drinking ourselves towards oblivion.

I gaze over the tinsel-bedecked computers and the streamers hanging from the ceiling. Alison has fed a Christmas compilation into a cassette player. The Band Aid single blasts over the desks. The younger staff have long-abandoned their tasks and are jigging, necking beer from bottles, slugging wine from plastic beakers.

Taking in the festive scene, I grin. The work we do is mundane, but we get along. There are cliques, and I'm not immune to this. I'm part of the smoking-room fraternity, where we gather and put the world to rights while immersed in a nicotine fug.

The managers will have seen my personnel file and appreciate why my position is probationary. Those who knew me when the office was based in Drumsheugh Gardens would have been aware of the mysterious weeks I was signed off. I've namedropped Andrew Duncan myself, the clinic typically associated with treatment for alcohol dependency rather than breakdowns. This was the plausible explanation.

Several colleagues have been skating the thin ice of the Scottish Office's drinking culture for years. Many crashing through. The extent of the latter ranges from bottles lolling around in drawers for topping up coffee, to an auditor who isn't averse to settling arguments by asking people outside. Some of the guys responsible for the archives, who operate mechanical carousels housing thousands of case files, are forever topping up the percentage proof of their bloodstreams. In Ghillies's. The Trafalgar. The Black Swan.

I think of working in Meldrum House in the months leading up to my second major hospitalisation. I would often join them in Mathers. One morning tea break offered an insight into their twilight world beyond the case files. A random woman marched over to the lad I'd just bought a pint for, lifted his glass and poured it over his head. Eighty bob dripping from his glasses, he just caught my eye, sniggered.

Another, Alistair, became a good mate. We were kindred spirits, veterans of the Royal Ed. Al had been studying botany at Uni but dropped out as his manic depression dipped. He would arrange to meet me in Tollcross for Saturday afternoon sessions. When I arrived at mid-day, he'd already be passed out in a corner. His lithium to lager ratio was several hundred milligrams beyond mine.

Unscrewing the second wine bottle, I fill a plastic cup to the brim. Watching the time creeping nearer noon, I open a Word document and jot some ideas for a short story.

A brilliant underground magazine was initiated on May Day this year, *Rebel Inc.* I attended the launch party, upstairs at James Thin's on the Bridges. In the wake of John Major's election win nine days earlier, its acerbic amalgam of fiction, poetry and interviews was showcasing the rising underground literary scene in Scotland. New writers were showcased over subsequent editions, many in print for the first time. Alan Warner. Sandie Craigie. Paul Reekie. Jenni Fagan. Barry Graham. Duncan McLean. Gordon Legge. Toni Davidson. John King. Irvine Welsh. And Anne's friend Laura Hird. Featuring slogans echoing punk fanzines: 'fuck the mainstream,' 'sharpasfuck fiction,' the journal epitomises 1992's countercultural zeitgeist. A lightning rod sparking in Scots. New editions are launched at riotous events soundtracked by DJ mixes, with raffle prizes including spliffs.

I know Sandie from the Gorgie/Dalry Writers' Workshop, held in the Adult Learning Project on the corner of Cathcart Place, two minutes from the flat. A charming woman from the Cowgate, we would chat about shared acquaintances from Edinburgh's punk scene as she fashioned her roll-ups. Her poetry is a glorious celebration of the local vernacular, perfect for the magazine's anti-Brit establishment vibe. I've had a couple of stories and poems rejected by their editor, Kevin Williamson, but I'm determined to get my name in there.

Over the years, I've accumulated enough of these letters to fill a ring-leaf binder, the majority predating my first breakdown. Right back to sending poetry that was an extension of my punk lyric writing to Riot Stories, the publishing imprint set up by Paul Weller when he was still in The Jam. This bulging folder is a testament, not just to my unpublished writing, but to the fragility of literary publishing in general. Many of the headed lettering is for long-vanished titles. *Edinburgh Review. Cencrastus. Panurge. Fiction Magazine.*

But rather than yet another pro-forma letter with a 'pp' signature, Kevin sent a handwritten A4 sheet, going into detail with suggestions to enhance my work. The key pointer: not to tell stories but show them through unique characters. To say this was inspiring would be an understatement.

So while the younger crew grow louder, their laughter ringing in my ears, I guzzle wine while my fingers type away. I've almost finished a draft of nine pages when word spreads that the first Joe Baksi has pulled in outside. I close the document without saving it.

*

In alcoholic self-destruct mode, I switch from wine to Diamond White cider after the meal. A cluster of these insidious green bottles is arrayed before me. The nearest has remained untouched for 15 minutes. Warning of an impending whitey. My attention flits to the dancefloor. Managers in paper hats shuffle to Wham's 'Last Christmas,' brandishing mistletoe at juniors ages with their daughters. I attempt a gulp. My throat recoils from what tastes like apple-scented battery acid. This sparks the fuse.

Snatching an empty pint tumbler, I bow my head beneath the table, coughing the bitter mouthful back. Eyes streaming, my guts feel like a washing machine in its final spin. Emptying the glass onto the carpet, I jump up and weave through all the leering faces to the sanctuary of the toilets. Claiming a cubicle,

I deep-breathe until nausea subsides. Rather than heading back into the clamour and brash disco lights, I blunder down the stairwell, two at a time, gulping at the icy air outside.

Staggering over Leith Street prompts a baying chorus of horns. The Scott Monument looming, I negotiate the crowds with difficulty, my vision revealing twice as many figures jolting past, driven by the desperation of securing last-minute gifts. As I stumble along, I realise I've left my overcoat. I'm shivering so much my thin suit now makes my mission to find an appropriate bus stop seem on a par with one of Napoleon's foot soldiers retreating from Moscow.

My homing instinct impels me to a bus stop, onto a Gorgie-bound 33. Taking a seat upstairs I find the warmth of the bus soothing. Queasiness wells again. Abates. My head rests against the window, dunting the pane.

*

My eyes flicker open. A moment of dumb incomprehension. Pain is boring into my eye sockets. I try retracing my day. Blank. Unfamiliar blocks of flats shoot past. Where am I? How did I get here? At the back of the bus, a youth is bragging about an act of violence, his mates cackling like hyenas. His rasping voice describes the noise a pool cue made cracking someone's skull. Panic lances through me. I ping the bell, exiting as the bus is still slowing, skiting along the pavement and crashing into the shelter.

It's snowing hard. My suit's fabric feels tissue-thin. I recall a TV advert about hypothermia that stressed the importance of wearing a hat because so much body heat escapes via your head. I tug the sodden purple tissue of the party hat I'm still wearing closer to my scalp.

Featureless scheme blocks stretch on all sides. Windows festooned with decorations are misty with warmth. Wind rushes past my face and howls through my hooped earrings. Within minutes, the storm intensifies until I can't see beyond the length of my outstretched arm. The bus stop's metal bar is like ice. Hands shoved deep into pockets, I shiver. I think of that advert again. Visualise a guy stumbling through snowdrifts, collapsing. Being wrapped in a thick tartan blanket by a rescue team who arrived by skis. Maybe a helicopter.

Time slows. My tears might freeze. Leaning against the perspex window my thoughts become delirious. It feels as if gravity has become a tractor beam sucking me towards the ground. Only sleep will release me from this nightmare. I slump onto the pavement. My head lolls. Tugging the collar of my jacket around my neck, I fold my arms. The world is sinking. The blizzard fades into a tranquil breeze wafting across a summer meadow. Bumblebees buzz around golden sunflowers.

My nose drips. My fist tightens around a hankie stuffed in a side pocket. When I tug out this ball of cloth, something else is extracted, spinning into the white landscape. I gaze after the mysterious object. A moment passes. I'm speared with alarm. Mustering some resolve, I heave myself up, balancing on my quivering legs. Layers of snow have caked the pavement, making it indistinguishable from the road. Bowing to my knees I burrow like a dog, fingers numbed to the pain.

A car races towards me, catches me in its dazzling headlights at the last minute. I scream. Somehow, despite the conditions, the driver avoids me, horn blast ringing. I hunker inside the shelter again, head bowed on my knees. I want to return to that meadow.

*

Someone is shouting. Snowflakes melt into my fluttering eye-lids. A minibus, a city sprinter, its headlights hurting my stare. The doors have opened to reveal the driver, a psychobilly with a resplendent bird of paradise hairstyle, peroxide quiff jut-ting. His shirt sleeves are rolled right up, revealing flourishing tattoos. Scottish saltires. Skulls. A bare-breasted woman with flame-red hair like something painted on the fuselage of a USAAF Flying Fortress.

When he demands I hurry up, I tell him I need to find something. I had a cassette. A C90. It's fucking vanished into the snow. Glowering, he tells me to forget it and climb aboard.

But I stress how important this tape is. Near hysterical. Scowling, he glances at the timetable pinned by his dashboard. Twisting the ignition key, he kills the engine. He rummages under his seat. Finds a torch. Now he eases into a leather jacket with an amazing tiger design etched into the back. *Where the fuck did you lose it?*

I stab my finger. He crunches across the uneven terrain, training the beam at the area I churned up. But his torch flickers then cuts out. *Fucking batteries*, he says, smacking it with the palm of his other hand. He extracts a Zippo, sparks a juddering flame. Shielding this from the howling wind, he glares at the ground. Clipping the lighter shut, he delves. Then he hands me the object. I blow the flakes away and dry it against my jacket. I'm euphoric. When he clambers back into his seat, I stagger behind, poking the C90 into an inside pocket.

I ask how much to Dalry? Fumbling into shrapnel, coins spill over the floor. He orders me to just take a seat before jerking in the ignition key, the diesel engine coughing. I slump into a chair behind him. Glancing over his shoulder, he asks my name. *Mark*. Pleased to meet you, Mark, he says. He's Larry. And a merry Christmas when it comes.

Heaving myself up, I lurch towards him, shaking hands. The vehicle's motion almost spins me down the aisle. He tells me to park my fucking arse, he doesn't want Eastern Scottish facing a lawsuit. But he insists I need to get straight home. Where is home? Springwell Place, I mumble.

He snaps about the fucking appalling death rate amongst the homeless at this time of year. Not to mention pissheads staggering home from office parties. My muttered thanks is so inadequate. Lightening the mood, he enquires what's so special about the cassette. So I tell him. It contains various recordings of my wee sister, Anne and me singing. Anne does 'Away in a Manger.' My party piece is 'Two Little Boys.' We're about seven and five. Another excerpt is me playing *Für Elise* on the piano, the last-minute practice before my Grade 1 exam that morning. My nerves were tempered with the knowledge of my reward for reaching this level: Dad taking me to my first football match in the afternoon, Hibs hosting Kilmarnock in the Scottish Cup 3rd round.

My dad taped these excerpts on a reel-to-reel recorder in the late Sixties; 1974 for the piano recital. Transferred everything to a cassette. *This* cassette. This is the *master* copy. The *only* copy. I'd taken it to work where a boy in the IT department was going to burn it onto a CD. But I found out he's off sick, so it stayed in my pocket.

When the bus lurches around a corner, I clutch a rail. I add that my dad also took a lot of cine footage, but they're silent movies. So this tape's the *only* recording of our childhood. Shrill voices frozen in time.

Fucking frozen, right enough, he muses. My eyes drift to his voluptuous redhead. Smiling at the fabulous story.

65

Sunshine On Edinburgh

August 2001

Dr Bowie asks why I felt the need to make this appointment. Distracted, she reminds me of someone. One of the Nostromo crew members massacred in *Alien*. And in *Witches of Eastwick,* she regurgitated cherry stones. By the hundreds. Veronica Cartwright. With a Tayside twang. There's a resemblance. Nothing like the doppelganger scenario during my depression.

I answer it's 10 years since I was discharged from hospital. At the time, my GP told me about lithium. He said my situation would be reviewed in 10 years. In case my circumstances had altered significantly. If, for instance, I'd settled down, with a family. I explain I got married last year. My wife Karen is expecting.

Although I bumped into Karen in Walkers, a West End nightclub, in the situation I met so many of the fading names in an address book, the chemistry was instant and overwhelming.

Glancing at my opened file on her desk, she mentions a stable relationship can have a positive influence on recovery. I broach the possibility of coming off my meds. I understood my lithium dosage would be reduced until such time I didn't need to take mood-stabilising drugs at all. And could lead a normal life.

Dr Bowie frowns. She wonders if I don't think I'm already leading a normal life? This, after all, has been the whole point of my being prescribed lithium. To maintain normality. What my GP suggested about my treatment being finite might have been his considered opinion. This didn't reflect the most recent research. Lithium stabilises patients who have experienced bipolar episodes but studies have shown patients coming off lithium have a 75% rate of regression. And when patients who have stopped taking lithium experience subsequent periods of mental ill-health, the episodes are *much* worse. The chemical imbalances that lead to certain people being more susceptible than others are mysterious. But what the psychiatric community are unequivocal about is that lithium can maintain stability.

After that barrage, I gaze at my case notes. Attempting to read upside down, I notice a yellow post-it. Scrawled in my handwriting. I ask her what it says? She studies the scrap, refers to the page: I handed this to a night nurse in Ward 1A during a bout of insomnia. Rotating the folder, she invites me to take a look.

It's weird skimming these clinical summaries. Dates. Medication dosages. Progress reports. Everything is in here. From the months leading up to the night Mum summoned paramedics who arrived with a police escort, through the psychiatric assessments and background, recommendations for rehabilitation, right up to outpatient treatment. I study the post-it.

My downstairs neighbour, May Annandale, was a nurse. Royal Army Medical Corps. She was one of the first females to enter Belsen after liberation.

The thought process that drove me to record that profound statement, then get up from my bed to hand it over to Ali, makes me smile. My bipolar compass was soaring in 1990. On another occasion, I became obsessed with contacting an ex, Louise. Convinced she was the lost love of my life and I had to propose to her by midnight before my 28th birthday to prove this. After a garbled phone call to the hairdressers where she once worked, a baffled colleague informed me she left ages ago and, as far as she knew, was now living in Cyprus. Waking in the morning, my recollection of that conversation was as embarrassing as the time I found God for 10 minutes.

Flicking through the file, I come across the typewritten statements by Dr Grant. Recommending upping medication doses. One catches my eye. June 1990. My parents should consider readmitting me as an inpatient. He mentions a carrier bag he discovered after my interview. Its contents are listed. A stash of Hibs programmes. A Scottish Ambulance Service badge. I recall Mum bought this from the YWCA shop in Henderson Row where she used to volunteer.

At the time, I was attempting to illustrate I was focused. Not crazed. Dr Grant's itemised list appears to confirm the latter. Forgetting to even mention the bag at the interview, I left it lying at my feet. After my admission to Ward 1A, he must've arranged to return it to Dad rather than risk stirring my already overactive mindset.

Turning the folder back around, I appreciate the symbolism. I'm accepting what experts in the field of psychiatric care are advising. To leave matters in their hands. That I'll always be reliant on my meds does seem a blow. I will never be 'normal' again. But people use prescribed drugs for myriad conditions. And what is 'normal'?

*

A crowd has gathered on the pedestrian precinct outside the Usher Hall. I spot a teenage girl sporting a Rangers shirt. My fluctuating interest in football means I'd choose music documentaries over watching it on TV. I might claim some lingering allegiance to her team when asked, although I've long been unable to name a single player and my final outing as a 'fan' was for their Scottish Cup victory over the old Airdrie nine years ago. On my last ever visit to Ibrox, for the preceding 4th round tie against Motherwell, my mate Jim and myself demolished a full bottle of Smirnoff on the train from Haymarket. Added to my medication, this resulted in me throwing up amidst the crowds thronging outside the stadium, then spending most of the match comatose in the Govan Stand toilets.

I think of how drinking with workmates could personify my bipolar swings. I picture Ghillies's, the bar in Trafalgar Street rammed every Friday, where guys would come round offering knock-off gear from holdalls containing everything from Armani jeans to steaks. One time, my vision swirling in a horrible combination of Carlsberg Special and lithium, I broke into an ugly chorus of 'God Save the Queen.' The fawning original that once contained the line 'Rebellious Scots to crush.' *Not* the vastly superior Sex Pistols version. My buddy, Mand dug an elbow to curtail my outburst, saving me from retribution in the staunch Hibs bar. She was the only workmate I ever confessed to about having been sectioned.

Scott Riddell was another close friend. An ardent Hibee, when we got drunk in Gladstones I would pronounce his surname like the high school in *Grease*, wrap my arm around him, and cajole him into joining me in Hibs anthems. *We are Hibernian FC. We hate Jam Tarts and we hate Dundee.* Eschewing partisan singalongs, he'd croon, *Would you like to swing on a star? Carry moonbeams home in a jar...*

He was such a sound guy. After one derby in Leith which Hibs won, as he was passing a couple of Jambos on his way home he said: *unlucky the day, lads*. He came into work on the Monday with a brutal black eye.

Scottie was also epileptic. Returning from the Gladstone toilets during one Friday payday session, there was an almighty crashing of glass. I assumed I was about to walk into a brawl and wondered if any of my company were involved. Scott was beneath an upturned table having a *grand mals* seizure. After his body ceased its horrible contortions, his line manager Andy caught my eye and shrugged. *Scottie fucking breakdancing again.* Scott suffered a fatal fit in his sleep. He was in his 20s.

Nowadays I've reverted to my first love, if the extent hasn't been anything more proactive than keeping an eye on their results – although I have given vent to that artistic streak rekindled in the IPCU. Karen and I run a craft website, 'SuperDoodles.' She receives orders to design Disney murals for nurseries and to paint portraits of pet dogs and cats. I create original football-themed birthday cards.

One example. A woman emailed to request a card for her husband, a lifelong Hibee, turning 60 last 16th January. I pored over dates from my Hibs reference books to find players and events sharing that anniversary. Amongst these volumes are several by John McKay, a Scottish Widows' actuary I once worked beside. I went on to source photos of the players referred to for the card's front, then added the relevant details to a table inside.

Jock Govan. 16.1.23. Son of a wounded WW1 veteran, born in staunchly Rangers Larkhall. Attacking full-back (decades before 4-4-2.) Playing behind Famous Five, won league champions medals 1951 and 1952.

Alex Cropley. 16.1.51. Tenacious midfielder and one of Turnbull's Tornadoes. Volleyed home 4th goal of 7-0 thrashing of Hearts, Ne'er Day derby in 1973.

Mickey Weir. 16.1.66. Winger, signed from Porty Thistle. In second spell at Hibs scored 25 in 158 appearances. League Cup medal in 1991.

16 January 1970. Scottish 1st Division. Hibs beat Aberdeen 2-1 at Easter Road. Goals by Pat Stanton and Joe Baker.

I've arranged to take samples to the Hibs shop to run by their promotions manager. I've also created cards for a Motherwell-supporting Church of Scotland minister, and through Anne, work colleagues supporting Celtic, Hearts, Bristol City, Sheffield Wednesday and Leeds United.

Through the throng, I can see a guy decorated with tribal tattoos, sporting a mohican, reminding me of Joe Strummer circa 'Know Your Rights.' He is enthralling everyone with a display of juggling flaming torches. Every so often he douses a torch by plunging it into his mouth. On other occasions, he spits paraffin to provoke a spectacular burst of flames. Dad used to perform the same trick in his loft workshop, mesmerising Anne and me.

Everyone alternates between gasps of astonishment and thunderous applause. These spectators represent people from all over the world, all age groups. Kids have been hoisted up to shoulder height for a better view of the fire-eater's escapades. Camcorders are trained on the performer. Cameras struggle to keep pace with his frenetic display.

As I spectate, I muse on the ups and downs of life. Lothian Road has hosted so many eclectic events over the years. Mum's older cousin Blanche was a member of the Young Communist League. She once described the day in 1934 when Oswald Mosley, the English fascist leader, held a meeting in that building beyond the whirring torches. His poisonous propaganda led to rioting in the streets outside, involving leftist protestors, and also supporters of John Cormack, leader of Protestant Action, an extremist sectarian group who commanded enough support to gain Edinburgh Council seats. So the night of the blackshirt rally there had been a three-way brawl typifying the perennial struggle between lumpen idiocy and the enlightened, involving anti-Jewish bigots, anti-Catholic bigots, and anti-bigots.

Fast-forward 30 years. Karen's mum, Alison was a modette in the 1960s, screaming to The Beatles, The Rolling Stones, The Hollies. I've seen performers as varied as Billy Connolly and Björk.

During the 1980s this part of central Edinburgh was brimming with bars and clubs and a focal point for pub crawls. For twentysomething bingers like I was, with an insatiable thirst for happy hour drinking, you could start at Tollcross and work your way north towards Princes Street, visiting a dozen pubs over the distance of a five-minute stroll. The return journey took a lot longer as you slalomed through an invisible assault course.

I ponder that although life will have downward spirals, will drag you to dark places, and if you are bipolar, can render you feeling worthless and suicidal, there is always a flip-side. Life may be a journey into the unknown, with so many unseen, unanticipated obstacles, but it's built into our DNA to focus on the light at the tunnel's end. To search for love and laughter.

This innate sense of optimism is unconnected to organised religion or half-baked life coaching. Faith and spirituality are existential terms so easily distorted, claimed, and exploited by individuals for their own ends. Analogous to those 19th-century land grabs when hordes of settlers rampaged across America's Midwestern prairies, emptied of their indigenous populations by European diseases the natives had no immunity from; or at gunpoint in the name of the Western culture and religion regarded as superior. Faith and spirituality are as core to humans as breathing. They have nothing to do with original sin or any of its variations across diverse sects or differing interpretations, equating to living under the perpetual threat of punishment in the next life. It's in the tangible euphoria experienced when we come together, communally, becoming one. Your team winning. Or being immersed in the sensory delights of music, whether you're amongst a dozen patients undergoing rehabilitation in a psyche ward, hundreds in a club, thousands at an open-air festival, or plugged into headphones and lost in your own playlist. Also, to paraphrase Kurt Vonnegut, in the silence following the final shot of a war.

It's in the simple chuckling face of the little girl next to me on her mum's shoulders, gazing at this show as if hypnotised by fire, the way humans have been for Millennia, as if these seconds unfolding before her are the most enthralling spectacle she could imagine. As John Lennon and Paul McCartney so succinctly put it. Love is all you need.

The fire-eater starts packing his equipment away and in a choreographed changeover, musicians emerge from the throng. Four lads with quiffs and brash Hawaiian shirts. Clutching bongos, a white guitar gleaming like a landed fish, and a double-bass festooned with stickers. The band assume position, not so much kick-starting their opening number as tearing into it as if they're speeding off their tits. They might well be. They're also radio-miked up to a small amplifier, channelling their immaculate harmonies, the clattering bongo beat reverberating back from the Grindlay Street tenements.

I clock their bassist, plucking at his strings as if they're red hot. Swivelling the instrument around in reckless circles. Red brothel creepers stomping the cobbles. Although any cockatoo hairstyle is bunched under a baseball cap, I recognise that face, chewing gum in time to the rhythm. The bus driver from the blizzard. Larry.

A few songs into their vibrant set, I ease my way closer, nodding along. When someone shifts position I find myself right at the front. I grin at the bass player. When he notices me, puzzlement for a second, then he beams. The breakneck song concluding with some nimble fretwork from the guitarist, Larry winks at his buddies. He announces, we're the West Side Comets. We're live at Teviot Row tonight, at 9 pm. Mark? Great to see you, buddy.

Heads crane in my direction. Larry continues, dedicating the next song to a cool guy he met one Christmas when he used to drive buses. He helped find some lost property for him. Something precious. The audience hangs on his every word. Larry persists. *Cool* was an understatement. It was a bitter December night when he discovered a guy in a suit partied out at a bus stop in the middle of Clovenstone. I was so blue with cold it was like Tom and Jerry.

Chuckles ripple through the assembly. He winks at me, tells his audience it might seem odd playing this on a beautiful summer's day, but it's *ironic*. Just like that Laurel and Hardy film, *Below Zero*, when they busk 'In the Good Old Summertime' in the middle of winter during the American Depression. This is like that, but in reverse. On this sunny August afternoon, in the company of all you beautiful people from all over the world, this is for you, Mark. It's called Ice Cold in Embra. *One Two Three Four...*

Grinning as these transitory moments of fame unfold, the communal clapping along to the rhythm rings in my ears. I notice a female rockabilly, auburn-haired, plaid shirt tight around her bare midriff to accentuate her curves, arms sleeve-tattooed. She might well be the inspiration for the ink on my saviour's forearm. This beauty is passing around a baseball cap spectators are already filling with change.

I pull my wallet out and open it. There, lodged behind the plastic window in its top compartment, is the image from Karen's three-month scan. Grainy, indistinct. But if you squint you can make out the profile. Not so long ago I would've thrust this towards her, explained that by saving my life her partner had played a role in creating this one.

Instead, I hand her a fiver. Beaming at me, she moves on. I glance at the photograph. I will spend the rest of my life trying to keep this tiny person safe.

66

Sunshine On Leith

May 2016

A gloriously sunny afternoon at Hampden Park, Glasgow. In the 2nd minute of injury time, 20-year-old midfielder Liam Henderson whips a corner into the Rangers box, captain David Gray connecting, heading past Wes Foderingham. The East Stand erupts, Hibernian's fans now nailbiting seconds away from witnessing the 114-year-old Scottish Cup drought vanishing. The final whistle is a cue for euphoric scenes.

So many emotions. I'm there with Karen's brother, Barrie and my nephews Ryan and Scott. All dyed-in-the-wool Hibees. The West Stand has thinned like a ruptured dam, the galleries muted by Antony Stokes' 80th-minute equaliser now silent. I appreciate some of the guys I used to watch Rangers with 25 years ago when my bipolar peaked, 20 years before the original club entered liquidation, may well have been amongst them.

Martin and his far-right FCS bullies. Ronnie, my wingman. Colin, who I sponsored for a skydive when my own head was in the clouds, days before being readmitted to the Royal Ed. This makes me think of Dr Grant's hand gestures. I touched 10 in the summer of 1990, my mental condition soaring with an incendiary cocktail. Dopamine. Alcohol. Cannabis. Before that, the long, dark autumn of 1987. Drowning in a remorseless whirlpool. Delusions. Agoraphobia. Insomnia. Nearing a state of madness by attempting to asphyxiate myself. Touching 0.

Flash-forward. Green and white bedecked hordes are streaming onto the pitch. I dwell on Dad taking me to my first Hibs match 42 years ago. Hating every minute of the experience as much as I loved every minute, he did so because that's what dads do. This brings tears. He would only have had a passing interest in today's result. But I wish he was there to answer the number still stored in my phone.

After he passed away two years ago, I would dial it now and again. Just to listen to his answer machine message. I imagine his affable Monaghan accent at least asking about the craic on this fantastic occasion.

*

Alan Stubbs becomes the first Hibs manager to brandish the Scottish Cup to the club's fans since 1902, the year before Grannie was born. This honour's previous holder was Dan McMichael (who eventually died from the Spanish Flu that infected one-third of the world's population after World War 1).

The massed choir breaks into 'Sunshine on Leith.' Thinking of 114 years, I fixate on another looming anniversary. This summer will mark 40 years since the Carberry Tower picnic.

I make a decision. The crime may be historic, but my assailant's description is ingrained in my damaged psyche. I can see him as vividly as if his face was looming through the swaying sea of green scarves. I've seen him since. Once. Driving through Gorgie with Karen and our daughter, Elise I glimpsed him pushing a wheelchair out of McDonald's. Seated, entrusting him with responsibility for her quality of life, was a woman around his age. Friend? Sister? Wife? When I was 13, I assumed he was a predatory gay man. He might just as easily have been a straight male for whom sexual predation was also about exerting power, a particularly abhorrent form of bullying.

I've already initiated detective work by tapping into the resource now utilised by professional crime agencies. *Facebook*. Through my own investigations, I've discovered Cairn Memorial Church, where the nonce lurked, faced the same situation as churches across Scotland, congregations dwindling in inverse ratio to spiralling upkeep costs, and were forced to merge with other local churches, becoming Gorgie Parish, and now Gorgie Dalry Stenhouse Church. I've already been trawling through photo galleries of cheery coffee mornings and folk concerts, searching for the man who derailed my 13-year-old life.

I make a resolution. After this weekend's triumphant events, and Karen, Elise and me have joined the throngs watching the open-top bus as it makes its way through Leith Links tomorrow, first thing Monday morning, I'm going to email

Lothian and Borders Police to request making a statement about being abused by a paedophile at a Church of Scotland picnic in 1976. But I dismiss the odious memories. Instead, I conjure a joyous vision.

Grannie, dancing to my band's first demo tape. Aged 78, swinging her arms to my jangly post-punk guitar. I imagine her being embraced by Grandad. Behind them, another couple. Her mother and her father in his Black Watch uniform, impervious to Flanders bullets, buttons gleaming, like the solitary photograph I've seen of him taken with his family, Grannie perched on her mum's lap.

In the background, Grannie's sisters, including Alice, a King's Theatre chorus girl, the first to burst into song at family parties, and Chrissie, asphyxiated in a carbon monoxide leak in her Portobello home.

Her niece, Blanche, mum's cousin, joins them. As a teenager, she loved dancing, from Fairley's in Leith Street to the Palais at Fountainbridge with its revolving stage and Tam Connery an occasional partner. I also picture Blanche's brother Billy. Clapping. A sapper, he fell in Normandy five days after D-Day. Aged 19.

Mum, an avid non-smoker who succumbed to lung cancer 11 years ago. Dancing with Dad. The horrible night of the ambulance long forgotten.

All of them, lost in music.